Intermittent Fasting for Women

How to Lose Weight, Boost Metabolism and Get Healthy

By Silvia Pala

**Copyright © 2020 Silvia Pala
All rights reserved.**

No part, portion or quotation exceeding 100 words in succession may be reproduced, copied or plagiarized in any way including being stored in a retrieval system or transmitted in any form or means such as photographs, screenshots, photocopying, recording, scanning, or other electronic or mechanical means, except those permitted solely under Sections 107 or 108 of the 1976 United States Copyright Act. Exceptions to this copyright can be given only upon written request for permission, granted by the Publisher. Such requests should be addressed to Silvia Pala, Servizi Linguistici, via Amilcare Ponchielli 1, 22063 Cantù (CO), Italy or via email to info@servizi-linguistici.com.

Limit of Liability and Disclaimer: Always consult your General Practitioner (GP) or primary caregiver before making decisions regarding your health. The author and publisher of this book make no claims to be held responsible for decisions you, the reader of this book, make regarding your physical and mental health. The author and publisher make no representations or warranties with respect to the completeness or accuracy of this work; however, they have published this book to the highest level of correctness and truth to the best of their knowledge. The warranty or guarantee of achieving a level of physical and nutritional fitness for any or all purposes is not made. The advice and strategies contained in this material may not be suitable for you, for example, if you suffer from any type of Diabetes or other physical or mental ailments. You should therefore always seek professional advice from your doctor, because this book does not warrant advice of a professional, legal, or medical nature. Any changes you make to your diet, lifestyle and state of mind should be made after one-on-one or another form of consultation with your primary care doctor, trusted physician or GP. Any reference to books, magazines, journalistic publications, websites or products has been made solely for the benefit of the reader. The author and the publisher have not and will not receive any gains from any means be it financial, in-kind, barter or gifts from any source, product, company, organization or institution mentioned or alluded to in this book. The information presented is purely for your benefit and not ours, in any way, and does not imply that the author or publisher endorses or is affiliated with the individual, organization, website, product or company mentioned herein. Readers should be aware that any websites or online materials referenced may not be available after the publication of this book, because the author and publisher do not take any liability for maintaining third party or external sources referenced.

Intermittent Fasting for Women: How to Lose Weight, Boost Metabolism and Get Healthy

Table of Contents

Introduction: 9
What is Intermittent Fasting? 9
Chapter 1: 11
Positive Effects and Benefits from Intermittent Fasting .. 11
    Weight Loss 11
    Muscle Gain 12
    Improved Fertility 13
    Reduced Inflammation 14
    Body Detox 15
    Reduced Stress/Hypertension 16
    Lower Cholesterol Levels 17
    Increased Longevity 17
Chapter 2: 20
Different Types of Intermittent Fasting Methods 20
    The 12 Hour Fast 20
    The 16 Hour Fast 21
    The 2 Day Fast (Otherwise known as the 5:2 Diet) 21
    Alternate Day Fast 22
    Weekly 24 Hour Fast (Otherwise known as Eat Stop Eat) . 22
    Meal Skipping 23
    The Warrior Diet 23
Chapter 3: 25
How to Track Your Progress as You Fast 25
    Keeping Track of Your Fast with Apps 25

Keeping Track with Smart Watches 26

Making use of Spreadsheets 26

Old Fashioned Pencil and Paper... 26

Chapter 4: **28**

Intermittent Fasting, Autophagy, and You **28**

    Here is a rundown of the known benefits of autophagy: **29**

    It Boosts Metabolism.. 29

    An Increased HGH Level.. 30

    Better Brain Health 30

    More Muscle Mass 31

    Reduced Inflammation 31

    Better Fat Burn... 32

    Increased Longevity 32

Chapter 5: **34**

What to Eat and Not to Eat During Intermittent Fasting 34

    What to Eat: **34**

    Coffee... 34

    Raspberries.. 35

    Low Calorie Beans and Legumes...................................... 35

    Blueberries 35

    Eggs 36

    Lean Chicken Breast 36

    Fish 36

    Veggies 37

    Whole Grains.. 37

    Yogurt 37

Dark Chocolate 37

Coconut Oil 38

What Not to Eat: 38

Soda 38

Heavily Processed Food 39

Sugary Sweets 39

Alcohol 39

Refined Grains 39

Trans-Fat 40

Fast Food 40

Chapter 6: 41

Additional Tips and Tricks to Ensure a Successful Fast. 41

Don't Get Bored 41

Satisfy Your Appetite with Zero Calorie Beverages 41

Don't Get Overwhelmed 42

Have a Good Attitude 42

Make Use of BCAAs 42

Fast While you Sleep 43

Use Proper Portion Control 43

Closely Monitor Your Results 44

Chapter 7: 45

Make Your Shopping List and Plan Your Meals Accordingly 45

Make Your Shopping List 45

Eggs/Dairy 45

Fruits/Veggies 47

Spices 49

Nuts/Legumes 49

Meat 50

Oils 50

Now Plan Your Meals Accordingly 51

For the 5:2 Method 52

For the 12 Hour Fast 53

For the 16 Hour Fast 54

For the Weekly 24 Hour Fast 55

Chapter 8: 56

Recipes of Suggested Dishes for Your Intermittent Fast 56

Breakfast Recipes 56

Indian Sweet Potatoes 56

Spinach and Scrambled Eggs 58

Quiche Breakfast Dish 59

Poached Eggs, Mushrooms, and Tomatoes 60

Cheesy Jalapeno Omelet 62

Sweet Potato and Egg Casserole 64

Lunch Recipes 66

Spicy Oven Baked Chicken 66

Lean Green Soup 67

Portobello Mushroom Fajita Wraps 69

Brown Rice Stir Fry 70

Low Carb Cabbage Bowl 72

Salmon and Green Beans 74

Carrot Topped Pizza 76

Seabass Fillets 77

Chicken Poblano Mix 79

Lean Beef Vegetable Soup 81

Tuna Fish Casserole Dish 82

Slow Cooked Spicy Chili 83

Snacks/Dessert 85

Sunflower Cookies 85

Homemade Dark Chocolate 87

Peanut Butter Bars 88

Low Cal Lemon Curd 90

Coconut Avocado Ice Cream 91

Fasting Snickerdoodle Cookies 92

Chia Seed Pudding 93

Refreshing Green Smoothie 95

Low Cal Cocoa 96

Dinner Recipes 97

Pineapple and Brown Rice 97

Chicken Vegetable Stew 98

Spicy Shrimp Stir Fry 99

Chickpeas, Tomatoes, Broccoli, and Spinach 101

Whole Wheat Spaghetti Dinner 102

Moroccan Orange Chicken Meal 104

Veggie Black Bean Burger 106

Beefy Maple Steak 107

Chapter 9: 110

The Recipe for Success: Balanced Diet, Sleep, and Adequate Exercise 110

Having a Balanced Diet 110

Getting the Right Amount of Sleep 111

Achieving Adequate Exercise 111

Chapter 10: **116**

Some Intermittent Fast FAQs **116**

Will Intermittent Fasting Make Me Fat? 116

What's the best time to exercise during a fast? 116

Would diet sodas be permissible during a fast? 117

Are there any initial negative reactions at the beginning of a fast? 117

Will I lose Muscle Mass during my Fast? 118

Do you have to spend much money prepping for your Fast? 118

Conclusion: **119**

Living Life in the Fast Lane **119**

Introduction:
What is Intermittent Fasting?

So, you've heard it before—just stop eating and you'll lose weight! Sounds easy enough right? Well, truthfully, it's really not. Because we humans you see, are creatures of habit and if we were to abruptly change our habits, like say suddenly not eat for three or four days, our bodies tend to get a little alarmed. In fact, rather than realizing that we're just trying to lose a few pounds to look good in a swimsuit—our body comes under the distinct impression that we are starving. Like literally, lost out in the wilderness somewhere, starving and about to die from a famine.

With all of these physiological alarm bells going off, the merciless hormones coursing through our system go on high alert and slow down our metabolism, as an emergency means of conserving our energy. This means that even while you're starving yourself to lose weight, your body is working against you double time to put that weight right back on! So, once you do start eating again; with your body in this hyper alert state of seeking to gain nutrients, whatever you eat will count twice as hard against you! Don't eat for a day and then suddenly that 200 calorie sandwich amounts to a 400-calorie sandwich! Not fair right?

Well, that's where intermittent fasting comes in, because intermittent fasting is a methodical approach to the same idea, except instead of a cold turkey fast, you fast in specific, pre-ordained increments. What's the difference? Well, if you fast one day for example, and then eat normally the next, your body is not as likely to slow down your metabolism. It helps to keep you on a more even keel. Since you are eating normally every other day, your body does not think that a sudden famine has struck the land, and will allow your metabolism to run at a more or less even clip.

At the same time, during your fast days, your system will get used to burning up extra fat, rather than calories. Fat you see, is the fuel reserve of the body. If you have extra fat hanging around your chest or waist, during a fast your body will start burning those fat deposits. Due to the lack of calories coming in, your system will automatically make use of the fat that already exists. Think of it like this, if you feel like the pizza you ate last week never quite left your body—well, when you fast, it finally will! Just allow your body to switch from burning carbs to burning fat and you can kiss those old fat deposits goodbye!

So it is that intermittent fasting brings you the best of both of these physiological worlds. You lose fat faster, due to a sudden drop in caloric intake forcing your body to burn up fat stores. But at the same time your metabolism shouldn't slow down since the eating routine remains stable every other day. Women the world over have come to see incredible results using just such a method. This is not hype—it's the truth. Because those who consistently fast within these parameters lose weight, boost their metabolism, detox their system, gain energy, and feel absolutely great.

If you agree, please leave us a review on Amazon after reading this book to tell us about your experience. Thank you for choosing this guide for your journey, and good luck!

Chapter 1:
Positive Effects and Benefits from Intermittent Fasting

Intermittent fasting can bring a wide range of positive effects and benefits. From burning fat to increasing energy and focus, all the way to the prevention of diseases and even the potential for greater overall longevity. To be sure, intermittent fasting isn't exactly easy. It requires a certain amount of patience, dedication and commitment. You have to arrange your schedule so that its conducive to the fasting routine—you must be mindful of what you eat and when you eat it. It's an adjustment that takes a little time to get used to. But for those that are willing to go the distance, the rewards are well worth the effort. Here in this chapter we will take a look at some of the most consequential positive effects and benefits that can be derived from intermittent fasting.

Weight Loss

Weight loss of course is the most sought-after effect of anyone on a diet, and intermittent fasting doesn't let you down. During a fast, the body goes through certain chemical reactions that induce it to start burning fat deposits rather than waiting for new calories to come in. In other words, since you are not eating, the body starts converting fat already in place on the body into readily useable energy. Insulin levels normally increase as we ingest food, but they lower when we fast. Decreased insulin signals the body that there is a lack of incoming nutrition, and that its time to switch gears and start burning fat instead.

Another chemical reaction that takes place has to do with something called "HGH", an acronym which stands for, "human growth hormone." Fasting increases these HGH levels dramatically, and it's HGH that streamlines the process of burning fat stores while also shielding us against muscle loss. Following on the heels of this recalibration, the nervous system begins delivering its special messenger of chemical change, "norepinephrine" to our fat cells. It is norepinephrine that then signals the fat to begin breaking down into what are known as "free fatty acids" that can be more easily catabolized as energy.

As you can see, due to the nature of the diet, the intermittent fasting gets the body running on all metabolic cylinders. After a day of fasting the body begins to eat away at fat stores and then the next day once you begin eating normally, the metabolism will pick back up where it left off, thereby allowing you to maintain the weight loss that you had achieved during your fast day. Keep this up for a long duration of time and you can lose a lot of weight. Not only that, you will lose weight in a much healthier way than would be the case in a near starvation diet. Because once again, it is the nature of intermittent fasting that helps to shield your body from metabolic extremes, keeping you on course for targeted fat burning for the long haul.

Muscle Gain

Intermittent fasting has the potential to not only maintain muscle, but to actually contribute to muscle gain. When the body goes through a period of fasting, several biological processes converge in an effort to conserve energy. As well as switching from burning incoming nutrients to burning fat deposits, the body also releases HGH (Human Growth Hormone) in an effort to conserve muscle building proteins. HGH works overtime to make sure that during times of extra stress and strain, your muscle's stay right where they are.

It's the pituitary gland that gives us HGH, and once released, this hormone only circulates for a few seconds before it is quickly made use of by the body. It still remains somewhat misunderstood, but there is indeed a direct correlation between the production of growth hormone and the body's ability not only to maintain lean muscle, but also to build it. HGH seems to help jumpstart this process.

Fasting increases the amount of HGH (Human Growth Hormone) that your body produces. Heavy consumption of carbs on the other hand, significantly reduces it. Through the process of intermittent fasting therefore, you can get your HGH back up and running and even gain a little muscle in the process. It is for precisely this reason some athletes actually take shots of HGH to improve their muscle production. But we don't have to buy an expensive shot of HGH from the doctor, we can simply produce our own from regular rounds of intermittent fasting.

Improved Fertility

It's true, intermittent fasting could indeed improve fertility rates among women. The human body you see, has a natural—built in—capability when it comes to allowing or hindering a woman's ability to get pregnant. This is why near starvation diets are bad. These kind of drastic changes in food intake make the body think that it is starving, and a time of famine is simply not a good time to get pregnant!

But having that said, intermittent fasting allows for the body to slim down and burn some fat while still keeping everything on an even enough keel to promote fertility. Intermittent fasting can even improve fertility levels by recalibrating the body's system during the fast/eat cycles. Even more intriguing, recent studies have shown that women who are dealing with complications from Polycystic Ovarian Syndrome (or as it is otherwise known "PCOS") can have their symptoms greatly reduced by engaging in regular intermittent fasting.

For women with PCOS, the periodic reduction in calories actually helps to fortify special "luteinizing hormones" that are crucial in regulating ovulation. In other words—it makes women more fertile, by having them produce eggs at more regular intervals. Intermittent fasting as it turns out is great at rebooting the system in a wide variety of ways and improved fertility is just another benefit gleaned from the overall results. Intermittent fasting makes for more streamlined ovulation. And the resulting improvement in fertility thereof, is just another proof of this wonderful recalibration process at work.

Reduced Inflammation

Inflammation is a natural reaction of the body's immune system when things are just a little bit unbalanced. If you happen to skin your knee for example, inflammation develops on the site of the injury to keep the wound from bleeding excessively and to clear out toxins. The resulting scab that a skinned knee produces, is a function of inflammation. Without the production of a scab by inflamed tissue, the wound would continue to bleed. In this situation, inflammation is obviously a good thing.

It is indeed a crucial function of our body, and it most certainly serves a purpose. But too much inflammation when it is not warranted can become a problem rather than a solution. Intermittent fasting can help clear up this chronic inflammation. It achieves this through the creation of something called "beta-hydroxybutyrate"—a natural beta-blocker that decreases the immune response when it comes to inflammation. This is good news for those that suffer from ailments such as arthritis and the like.

During intermittent fasting beta-hydroxybutyrate is released and immediately begins work blocking certain receptors of the immune system that are responsible for inflammation. And it's the powerful immune receptor, the so-called "NLRP3 inflammasone" in particular that beta-hydroxybutyrate immediately latches onto and subdues its inflammatory response.

Again, inflammation is a natural response of the body, and in some cases is necessary. Chronic inflammation however, leads to such things as arthritis and hypertension. In today's world, much of the food we eat is overly processed and loaded with carbohydrates.

This my friends, is simply a recipe for unwarranted and out of control inflammation. Intermittent fasting however, allows the body to scale back this process and reduce unnecessary inflammation.

Body Detox

Intermittent fasting puts the body through a process called "autophagy." The term literally means "self-eating." As strange as it might sound, it's a very beneficial process in which the body seeks out damaged or dead cellular material, consumes this excess junk, and then spits it back out as brand new healthy cells. In other words, it's a process by which we can detox.

Autophagy is a routine process that occurs all the time, but typically at a much slower rate than it does during periods of fasting. Intermittent fasting kicks autophagy into high gear however, and allows your body to detox itself of toxins, waste, dead cellular debris—you name it, at a much faster pace. Intermittent fasting shifts the body from burning carbs to burning fat, and in so doing, it also automatically kickstarts the process of autophagy as well.

You may now be noticing a theme in this book, that seems to touch upon every aspect of intermittent fasting. Fasting at its core, is a practice that sends the body into a kind of standby mode in which vital processes are kept running by conserving and making use of material that is already available. For us humans, that material is our stored fat, as well as cellular debris.

By using fasting to get ourselves into this stasis state we reap the benefit of burning up fat stores as well as detoxing our system of needless cellular waste. Like a clean-up crew suddenly summoned to aisle 2—autophagy mops up the mess and gets the ball rolling. If you really want to detox put down that fruit juice and pick up intermittent fasting instead!

Reduced Stress/Hypertension

A steady regimen of intermittent fasting could very well lower your blood pressure. In fact, according to a recent study that appeared in an edition of "Nutrition and Healthy Aging" back in 2018, noted that among 23 test subjects, those who engaged in a regular intermittent fast experienced a decided drop in blood pressure.

As noted earlier, a leading cause of hypertension is an overabundance of inflammation in the body. And as mentioned, intermittent fasting helps to reduce that inflammation. In addition to this, intermittent fasting has also shown itself to be a direct factor in the reduction of stress and hypertension. An intermittent fast lowers insulin levels, and with it, both symptoms of hypertension and stress are considerably eased.

Most probably think of stress as "mental stress" but in reality, our bodies face stress all the time on a holistic level through what is termed "oxidative stress." And more often than not, this biological oxidative stress when in over abundance, can lead to psychological stress. Many patients suffering from anxiety, depression and the like have been found to have inordinately high levels of oxidative stress in their cellular makeup. Intermittent fasting helps to shield our body's cells from undergoing too much oxidative stress by reducing the incidence of harmful molecules called free radicals in the body.

Free radicals are molecules that are highly unstable and contain "highly reactive electrons." It's these free radicals that bounce around the body bumping into other molecules and disrupting their own charge. This in turn creates a domino effect in which the disrupted molecules themselves become free radicals and as the collateral damage adds up, it leads to tremendous oxidative stress on the cells of the body. Free radicals often originate from faulty mitochondria within our cells.

And as mentioned earlier into this book, it is the detoxifying state of autophagy that cleans house and gets rid of such faulty cellular material, thereby preventing the rise of free radicals. Which in turn reduces oxidative stress. Oxidative stress is no joke and can cause a wide variety of problems. But autophagy gets right to the root of the problem, this then reduces stress and hypertension as a whole—all across the board.

Lower Cholesterol Levels

While more research still needs to be done—studies have indeed shown that regular intermittent fasting has the propensity to lower that "bad cholesterol" known as LDL, which stands for "low-density lipoproteins". These lipoproteins are responsible for bringing our cholesterol levels to unhealthy heights, but intermittent fasting can greatly reduce their prevalence. In fact, recent research has indicated that out of study participants who engaged in intermittent fasting over a period of roughly 3 months, managed to cut down their LDL by as much as 25 percent.

There has been some argument in recent years over whether or not those who have high cholesterol should engage in intermittent fasting. And to be sure, if you have high cholesterol, be sure to consult your doctor before starting an intermittent fasting regimen. But as these recent studies have shown, if done properly, long term intermittent fasting could indeed have the capacity to significantly lower cholesterol levels.

Increased Longevity

Did we mention that intermittent fasting can help you live longer? Yes, if nothing else—intermittent fasting might actually help you live longer! There have been many studies recently that have shown the benefits of caloric restrictions. Mice that have been subjected to an intermittent fast for example, have been shown to actually live longer.

So, if you think that eating those microwaveable hot pockets every lunch break is killing you—you just might be onto something! Because our heavily processed foods, loaded with carbohydrates are not only making us fatter, but also increasing the disruption posed by free radicals, creating oxidative stress, and producing unbearable inflammation. Intermittent fasting could be a cure for all of these things and as a result could very well increase your longevity. As you can see, there are more than enough reasons to give intermittent fasting a try. So, what are you waiting for?

A Look at the Long History and Appreciation of Intermittent Fasting

The recent popularity of intermittent fasting can be credited to Dr. Michael Mosley, a regular contributor to the BBC who in 2012 created a documentary on the subject called "Eat Fast, Live Longer" which highlighted the benefits of the practice. But although it was Dr. Mosley who recently brought intermittent fasting into the spotlight, it's by no means new. Intermittent Fasting in fact, actually has quite a long history in practice.

It could be argued even, that by our very nature, humans are hardwired to go through periods of feast, as well as famine. This all dates back to our prehistoric ancestors who rather than settling down in one spot and growing crops, were more apt to be hunter gatherers. This meant that in order to have a meal they had to go find one first, and when there was simply nothing to hunt and nothing readily available to gather, they did without. This had our bodies conditioned to take in calories when they were available but also learn how to live off of extra fat deposits when they were scarce.

It was under these conditions that intermittent fasting was born. And even after folks settled down into agricultural communities where food was grown and stored year-round, fasting continued.

Many religions in fact such as Judaism, Christianity, Islam, and even Hinduism, all have fasting as a part of the religious experience. The reason? Along with displays of faith and dedication, fasting tends to bring more focus to mind and body and ostensibly thereby bring one closer in their connection with God. Even if you aren't particularly religious however, these same qualities of attunement and focus in life brought on by fasting can still be appreciated.

Chapter 2:
Different Types of Intermittent Fasting Methods

Perhaps the greatest allure of the intermittent fast is how flexible it is. Because truth be told, there isn't just one way to fast—there are several ways to fast. You may have heard of the 5:2 diet, or perhaps the 12 Hour fast? But maybe alternate day fasting is more your style? It's entirely up to you. Depending on your schedule, you can create fasting patterns that work best for your own personal routine. If for example, you tend to eat light during the work week but then eat your way through the weekend—no problem! There are fasting regimens designed for you! On the other hand, if you would like to fast one day and then eat normally the next in rapid succession, there is a fasting regimen for that as well. Here in this chapter we will go over all of the many different types and methods that can be employed when it comes to intermittent fasting.

The 12 Hour Fast

There are only 24 hours in a day, and we all go about our business one 24 Hour cycle at a time. This fast has the participant fasting for half of that 24-hour allotment. Considering the fact that a healthy night's sleep consists of anywhere between 7 to 9 hours, the time you sleep could be part of the time you fast. Having that said, let's say for example that you went to bed at midnight and woke up at 7 in the morning. Well—congratulations! This means that you've already fasted for 7 out of your 12 hours! Good job!

That was pretty easy, huh? Now in order to complete your 12 Hour Fast, all you have to do is refrain from eating over the next 5 hours. That means your 12 Hour fast would end at 12 noon. In that case, fasting from midnight to 12 noon is essentially just skipping breakfast. While this may seem like a bit of a lightweight challenge for some of the more hardcore adherents to fasting, it still does indeed do the work of priming the body to burn fat. Even while you sleep you see; you can get your metabolism to turn on the body's fat burners.

The 16 Hour Fast

Working on the same premise as the 12 Hour fast, the 16 Hour fast simply extends the fasting window by 4 additional hours. Fasting for 16 hours rather just 12 can get the body to begin burning up fat stores at a much faster rate. Similar to the example above of someone who fasts from midnight to 12 noon, in the 16 Hour fast, the fasting could be extended all the way until 4 PM that evening. This means skipping both breakfast and lunch, in favor of simply having an early evening meal. Many have sighted this fast as not only helping them burn fat, but also as providing a much more enjoyable evening routine as they round off their day with a well-deserved, satisfying evening meal. If anything else, you won't have to figure out what to make for breakfast and lunch since both fall within your fasting periods. With this fasting strategy, all you really have to do, is just eat a good dinner and let your metabolism do the rest.

The 2 Day Fast (Otherwise known as the 5:2 Diet)

As was mentioned earlier, if you tend to be less mindful of your eating habits during the week than you are on the weekend, then the "2 Day Fast" or as it is otherwise known, the "5:2 Diet" just might be for you. This plan has the dieter eating normally for 5 days of the week but either directly fasting, or at least reducing caloric consumption to under 500 calories, for 2 days. Some who employ this fasting method tend to sandwich their fasting days in between their eating days.

If for example, they eat on Monday, they then fast on Tuesday, and then if they eat on Wednesday, then they fast on Thursday—finishing up the cycle by once again eating normally on Friday and the weekend. Others however who wish to eat normally during the work week, might be tempted to simply fast their 2 days full force, right at the end of the week, during the weekend when they can take the time to be more mindful of their routine. Either way works fine, it's just a matter of what works better for the person who is doing the intermittent fast.

Alternate Day Fast

Alternate Day Fasting works on a similar premise as the 2 Day Fast. Because like the 2 Day Fast in which someone could eat one day and fast the next—the Alternative Day Fast works on this premise as well. The Alternate Day Fast takes things further however, because instead of just two fast days the adherent to this regimen will have three fast days. This means that if someone eats on Monday, they then fast on Tuesday, they eat on Wednesday, they then fast on Thursday, they eat on Friday, they then fast on Saturday and eat on Sunday—so on, and so forth.

Some consider this regimen to be a bit "extreme" but in many ways it is quite successful because it relies on the full concept of intermittent fasting. This method allows someone to fast for a full day, buttressed by full feeding days in between which prevent the body's metabolism from dramatically slowing down. This is great for someone trying to lose weight because while their body is benefiting from fat burn during the fast days, their overall metabolism will not be affected as long as they choose to eat normally during every single day between their fasts. All in all, it's a guaranteed win-win situation. If this sounds like a program that would work for you, don't hesitate to give it a try.

Weekly 24 Hour Fast (Otherwise known as Eat Stop Eat)

For those that wish to take part in the "Weekly 24 Hour Fast" or as it is sometimes known the "Eat Stop Eat" diet—you must be prepared to eat absolutely nothing for 24-hour intervals. For some who get a little shaky from not eating for several hours at a time, this may be a little bit of a shock to the system. Such prolonged fasting after all could cause feelings of exhaustion, irritability, headaches, and a few just might get a little hangry (hungry and angry) about the whole ordeal.

In all seriousness, it's not exactly the easiest means of intermittent fasting, and is only recommended for the some of those hardier souls out there, who are up for a challenge. It's definitely not for everybody, but for some however, who like to go all or nothing, it could be the best fasting strategy for them. Also, if you are already used to fasting, your body should more or less adjust to it. It's for this reason that the 12 hour and 16-hour fasts are often stepping stones that help one work their way up to a full 24 hour fast. It's all a process after all, and works for one may not work for others. There is no one size fits all. So feel free to experiment.

Meal Skipping

Never you mind what your mother may have told you, skipping meals could be sometimes alright. The "Meal Skipping" fast—just like it sounds, is a fast that involves routinely skipping meals. This could be a good fasting routine for someone that is just starting to experiment with denying their bodies of food. Meal skipping can be as easy as skipping lunch, breakfast, or dinner. This method of fasting helps individuals to eat when they are hungry and then opt out when they are not. Although it does not necessarily bring in the most dramatic results when it comes to weight loss, meal skipping does help one become more in tune to their own physiological needs. And it lets them learn to know when they are really hungry in the first place, rather than simply grazing, or engaged in a bout of mindless eating.

The Warrior Diet

Do you feel like a warrior? Do you like a challenge? Then you just might want to try "The Warrior Diet." This diet takes your 24-hour window and shaves your main eating time down to just 4 hours. Under this regimen the rest of the 20 hours of each and every day is spent fasting from most foods, with the exception of eating small amounts of fruits and veggies. Like usual, the main goal on a fast day for this method, is to keep your caloric consumption under the 500-calorie limit.

The Warrior Diet allots only one main course meal for the dieter, during a finite 4-hour window. Many save their 4 hours for the end of the day, allowing them to have at least one satisfying evening meal after fasting most of the day. It is recommended that during the 4-hour feeding window, participants should load up on plenty of healthy carbs. Under this routine you've got just 4 hours to eat the food you really like so you better make it count!

Feel free to try any and all of the fasting routines mentioned in this chapter until you find what's right for you.

Chapter 3:
How to Track Your Progress as You Fast

We live in a world that is constantly in motion and we have become accustomed to tracking many aspects of our lives. We routinely track financial transactions, we track our location through GPS, and we even track how many steps we might take on any given day through our Fitbit. But how do you track your progress as you fast? Regardless of what fasting method you may choose, you are going to want to track your progress so you can stay within your goals, and make adjustments if necessary. Being able to monitor your fast in real time will serve as a great morale booster as you take note of how far you have come. And there are quite a few ways that this can be done. Here in this chapter, we will explore some of the options available.

Keeping Track of Your Fast with Apps

Yes, there is an app for that. For a more modern approach, there are some excellent apps for tracking the progress of your fast such as the "MyFast" app currently available on Google Play and the App Store. Referred to as an "intermittent fasting management" application—this app allows you to plan out your whole schedule through a digital calendar that you can customize and edit at any point during your fast, in real-time. Yet another popular app for intermittent fasting is the "BodyFast" app.

This app touts itself as working like an "individual coach." It is geared to help you determine the best intermittent fasting method, according to your own schedule and immediate goals. It does this by factoring in various personal information into the app so that it can coach you on the best routine. If you are having a hard time deciding the best course to follow in your intermittent fasting—

BodyFast could indeed be a good app to use. There are also many calculating apps available online. One of the best of these is "Vora" which can link right up to the cloud to store your data.

Keeping Track with Smart Watches

Smart watches such as the Apple Watch and the Samsung Galaxy Watch are currently all the rage. They can do just about anything your phone can, and they can also be of use in tracking your progress as you fast. Just program the info in your watch's calendar and allow the built-in programming of your watch to take over. The Apple Watch for example, has fitness programs that take stock of your own personal circadian rhythm so that you are able to track fasting even while you sleep. The watch is currently geared to support 18-hour fasts, 20-hour fasts and even 36-hour fasts. If you don't have one already, put it on your wish list, because it's a great tool to have at your disposal, for this and a wide variety of other reasons.

Making use of Spreadsheets

Some may roll their eyes at the notion of keeping track of their progress in a spreadsheet. But if you don't have access to apps or a smart watch, another easy way to keep track of your fasting routine would be to use a spreadsheet. Most computers come with spreadsheet software already installed. Microsoft Excel from the traditional Microsoft Office Suite should work just fine. Just plug your fasting data into the electronic spreadsheet and update the information as you progress through your fast. Even if you have never used a spreadsheet before, they are relatively easy to learn. There are also plenty of tutorials out there to help teach you along the way. It may not be the fanciest means of keeping score, but it will certainly get the job done.

Old Fashioned Pencil and Paper

If all else fails—if your apps fail to download, your computer crashes, or you lose your smartwatch—just pull out an old-fashioned pencil and piece of paper! It may sound a bit quaint, but trust me it works. Just draw a small chart for yourself and use it to list the days of your fast. Keep your entries in a safe place and continue to consult them as you track your progress. Even notes scrawled on a piece of paper will serve as a great reminder of the milestones you have achieved during your intermittent fast. At any rate, however it is that you decide to do it, always be sure to track the progress of your fast.

Chapter 4:
Intermittent Fasting, Autophagy, and You

Many have come to realize that intermittent fasting packs a powerful punch when it comes to weight loss and overall health. But precious few understand the innerworkings that facilitate such powerful results. The real engine under the hood when it comes to intermittent fasting, is the process of autophagy. As mentioned earlier in this book, autophagy—which literally means "self-eating"—is the process of the body eating up and disposing of toxins, dead cellular debris, and other useless waste material in the body.

Autophagy is the body's means of cleaning out old junk that it no longer has use for. This includes wasted protein, shed cell membranes, and discarded cellular components called organelles, along with defunct mitochondria. But the process of autophagy doesn't just toss these things to the side, it recycles them, and refurbishes dead cellular material into new cellular components. Absent of autophagy, the other way that the body gets rid of old cells is through the pre-programmed cell death of apoptosis.

In apoptosis however, cellular material isn't recycled, it's simply written off for good. The cellular environment gets too crowded, so some cells naturally have to be liquidated. This is precisely what happens with someone who has tissue that is chronically inflamed. When too many cells are in the neighborhood, some of them will have to be forced out of the picture through programmed cell death, it's as simple as that. But when the body is forced to quickly kill off overabundant cells, it leaves behind a lot of cellular waste.

In this vicious cycle, this buildup of junk, can actually contribute to even more inflammation as the body seeks to clear this debris out. Autophagy is more beneficial than apoptosis in the sense that rather than creating more waste, it is utilizing material that already exists in order to create new cells. In this process, there is no need for a massive inflammatory response from the body, and since waste material is used to refurbish cells, the process is streamlined and bodily tissue is much stronger for it.

Since outside nutrients are not as forthcoming during a fast, the body begins to turn inward and literally consume itself—at least it's more expendable members—in order to maintain energy. In much the same vein that fasting causes the body to burn fat for fuel, it also revs up the part of recycling old and damaged pieces of cellular material into new, healthy, and more streamlined cells. This process has been championed as being beneficial for the prevention of many diseases—and has even been touted as capable of even reversing cancer. But don't just take my word for it. Let the facts speak for themselves.

Here is a rundown of the known benefits of autophagy:

It Boosts Metabolism

Autophagy provides a decided boost to metabolism. And if you don't believe me—then perhaps you might believe the folks down at the NCBI (National Center for Biotechnology Information), who wrote up a recent report stating that autophagy was, "a powerful promoter of metabolic homeostasis at both the cellular and whole-animal level." In other words, it gets your metabolism started in a hurry.

Metabolism itself if you think about it—is the rate at which the body burns up nutrient resources. If there isn't a steady stream of nutrients coming in from the outside, as would be the case when fasting, the body then has no choice but to turn inward. The fast will eventually trigger the process of autophagy, which has the body gobbling up toxins, waste products, and dead and/or defective cellular debris. All the junk is cleared out so new cells can form.

It will also serve to generally speed up the metabolism in the process. As autophagy cleans out old mitochondria for example—the part of the cell that burns through fat stores—and replaces them with new ones, it is as if the very motor of your body's cell has been overhauled, primed and tuned up, allowing for a much smoother ride when it comes to your body's metabolic rate. So, get ready to go full throttle, because autophagy most certainly does boost your metabolism.

An Increased HGH Level

As mentioned earlier in this book, human growth hormone plays a critical role when it comes to intermittent fasting and the ability of the body to quickly and efficiently lose weight. Human growth hormone is also an important factor in play when it comes to autophagy. Autophagy helps to produce HGH. And as it turns out, once that said HGH is processed by our liver, it in turn reinforces and contributes to the autophagy already present. So, what you end up with is a complete, positive feedback loop of a steady state of autophagy. The body will then be able to much more rapidly heal and build new tissue. You see, there's a reason why athletes spend a fortune to get HGH shots. If a football player past their prime needs a boost, they just might invest in HGH. But thanks to intermittent fasting you won't have to pay a dime! Just stick to your selected fasting routine and your HGH levels will increase naturally.

Better Brain Health

I used to work in an office for a guy who was rather fond of reminding his employees that a cluttered desk is the sign of a cluttered mind. This may have just been a pep talk to get us to clean our desk, but he probably didn't realize just how cluttered people's minds could truly get—and it had nothing at all to do with poorly kept office space. Because our brains do indeed get cluttered. Over time, they become cluttered up with dormant proteins and other unused material lodged between the cells that makes up our brain.

The process of autophagy is useful in snatching up these latent proteins, repurposing them for energy, and getting them out of the way. Even for those with serious degenerative conditions such as Alzheimer's, a good round of autophagy has shown promise in clearing out the "amyloid" protein which is a primary contributor to the condition. Clearly, more research needs to be done, and no one is saying that autophagy is a clear-cut cure for serious degenerative conditions. Having that said however, there is a clear correlation between this process and improved cognitive function. Yes, your brain does indeed benefit from autophagy. Our minds can apparently become pretty cluttered and its autophagy that works to clean house.

More Muscle Mass

As we get older, we are all more prone to losing some of our muscle mass. But there are ways that we can proactively prevent the onset of muscle loss. Regularly working out of course, is a big help, but it doesn't always do the job. The process of autophagy however, can work to improve your muscle mass from the ground up. It's in fact, a decided lack of autophagy which contributes to age related muscle loss in the first place. So, having that said, a good fast every now and then, just to get the autophagy afterburners going, could indeed keep you from losing too much muscle mass in the future. So just keep this in mind. Autophagy can keep you looking your best. And if you want more muscle mass—all you really have got to do is *fast-fast-fast*, and autophagy will do the rest!

Reduced Inflammation

Inflammation is a natural response of the body to stress. It may not sound like it, but in certain situations, this inflammation can be a good thing. If you sprain your ankle for example, the resulting inflammation is necessary to begin the process of healing. But at other times, chronic inflammation as is experienced with something such as arthritis is a decidedly bad thing. The process of autophagy, as it turns out, can stop inflammation right in its tracks. It does this by eliminating the proteins known as "antigens" which are known to cause inflammation to erupt in the first place. By keeping antigens at bay, autophagy can significantly reduce any and all inflammation that someone may experience. This is good news for those suffering from arthritis and other inflammatory conditions.

Better Fat Burn

As mentioned in the previous section, autophagy can help to reduce any inflammation that may be present in the body. This reduction in inflammation could also be key to losing weight, since lowering inflammation, also lowers insulin, which is a known factor when it comes to the body hanging onto fat deposits. Lower insulin means less fat storage and weight loss. Autophagy trains your body to store less fat. But of course, the most immediate means through which autophagy burns up the fat is by revving up our metabolism and getting rid of waste products outright.

Increased Longevity

As mentioned earlier in this book, intermittent fasting seems to show promise in enhancing longevity. And autophagy is most likely an important factor in this process. In several studies now, lab rats have been induced into states of autophagy, and all have been shown to live longer and to be in "better overall shape." Admittedly studies conducted on mice, may not be the most appealing when it comes to human beings. But if autophagy is capable of enhancing the life of lab rats, it should also be able to enhance the lives of people too. Yes, if anything else, autophagy just might help you to live longer. And that's certainly something to be happy about.

To be clear, autophagy is a natural process that occurs in all of us, all the time. But it typically occurs at a much slower rate than it would while we are fasting. And it is said that autophagy really kicks it into high gear after fasting for at least 20 hours straight. This is the threshold for autophagy and thereafter the body begins to quickly burn through defective cellular debris and loose proteins in order to make up for the lack of nutrients. Having that said, a straight fast such as during the "weekly 24 hour fast" mentioned earlier in this book would be ideal for those wishing to benefit from autophagy.

Chapter 5:
What to Eat and Not to Eat During Intermittent Fasting

No matter how you plot your path when it comes to an intermittent fast, you need to have an understanding of what is good to eat, and not eat during your efforts. Unless you are engaging in a complete fast from solid foods for 24 hours, you will have to know just what you should eat on your fast days. Likewise, it would be good to know what might be best suited for your non-fast days too. Because remember, just because you might be on one of your non-fast days, doesn't mean it would be a good idea to go downtown and binge at the all you can eat buffet. Here in this chapter we will help guide you to make wise food choices on what to eat and what not to eat during your intermittent fasting.

What to Eat:

Coffee

Okay, well it's not really a food, but coffee as a zero-calorie beverage is a great supplement to any fast day. Most of us can't do without a cup of coffee in the morning as it is, so this is most certainly good news for those of us who enjoy our cup of morning joe. Coffee can also help to ameliorate possible negative reactions to fasting. If your initial fast has you feeling a bit lethargic and lacking in energy for example, a good stiff cup of coffee could certainly help to offset those symptoms. But keep in mind that the coffee needs to be taken straight out of the pot, foregoing any creams or sugars. For some of you, unsweetened coffee just might have to be an acquired taste, but if you ditch the sugars and creams, you will be a lot better off in the long run.

Raspberries

Raspberries are a low-calorie food that won't wreck your fast day and at the same time, will help keep you regular by giving you healthy dose of fiber. Raspberries also come replete with healthy vitamins and minerals, as well as inflammation busting antioxidants. This is good to ward off arthritis and other degenerative conditions. In some situations, raspberries are even said to prevent cancer. This is due to a powerful cancer busting phytochemical it boasts, called "ellagic acid." At any rate if you have nothing else to eat on a fast day, bowl of plain, simple, raspberries would be a good dietary choice to make.

Low Calorie Beans and Legumes

Beans, beans, the magical fruit. The more you eat, the more fat you can burn for your fast. Both beans and legumes are packed with healthy nutrients and are typically low in calories. They also have plenty of protein, helping to keep your muscles fueled even while your fat stores are depleted. Tiny but mighty, beans and legumes are fully capable of aiding in the process of weight reduction, during your intermittent fast. Most especially good when it comes to intermittent fasting are peas, black beans, lentils, and garbanzo beans.

Blueberries

These fruitful treats are low in calories yet high in antioxidants, helping to ensure the body remains free of nasty free radicals that could degrade bodily tissue over time. Blueberries are known immune boosters too, good for ensuring you don't get sick or otherwise compromised while you fast. Another neat thing about blueberries is that they contain a little something called flavonoids, which if consumed over a long period of time, can work to reduce overall BMI (Body Mass Index). This is most definitely a good thing. And did I mention? They also taste great!

Eggs

Whether you hard boil them, scramble them, or poach them—the incredible, edible egg is a great low calorie, nutrient dense food for your fast days. Eggs just seem especially geared for this task. Eggs have a ton of proteins and tend to stick with you, leaving you filling full and satisfied. If you are indeed allowing a small allotment of under 500 calories on your fast day, adding a couple of eggs to the mix certainly won't ruin your fast.

Lean Chicken Breast

If you aren't doing a 24 hour fast, a serving of lean chicken breast is a good way to end a fast day that shouldn't exceed your 500-calorie allotment. Lean chicken breast provides plenty of proteins without all the filler of other sides of meat. It's also a mainstay that goes well with quite a few meals and recipes. Here, in this book for one, you will find plenty of dishes that make full use of the power of a piece of lean chicken. Having that said, you should definitely stock up on some lean chicken breast in preparation for your next intermittent fast.

Fish

Just like chicken, fish is a good source of protein and yet won't break your budget of allotted calories on your fast day. Fish has a ton of what are known as omega-3 fatty acids. Don't let the "fat" word scare you thought, because omega-3 fatty acids are a good thing. There's a reason why every health food store has aisle after aisle of omega-3 supplements. Because its omega-3 fatty acids that can safeguard our heart, dramatically reduce blood pressure, clear out plaque from arteries, and even prevent heart attacks and strokes. Fish is also considered a "brain food" due to its ability to help enhance cognitive function. Fish—it's decidedly nutritious, and it's downright delicious! Be sure to make use of it.

Veggies

You don't have to be a vegetarian to appreciate the tremendous benefit that veggies can provide. Vegetables represent a stabilizing force on your non-fast day and every day between. As well as providing plenty of valuable nutrients, veggies also give us a healthy dose of fiber to help keep us regular. Vegetables are typically low in calories too, so you can mix and match them with all kinds of meals regardless of meal plans. Be sure to have plenty of fresh veggies on hand.

Whole Grains

Whole grains are a great source of nutrition on fast or non-fast day either one. Unlike refined grains that spike your insulin, these morsels won't make you mess up your fast, and will still leave you feeling full and satisfied. You will find quite a few recipes in this book that make use of whole grain. It makes for a good bread alternative, so if you are ever in doubt—just reach for the whole grains!

Yogurt

When people think of health foods, one of the first things that come to mind is probably yogurt. Yogurt is an excellent source of nutrients and also provide a boost to your metabolism and energy even as you fast. Yogurts also come complete with a dose of probiotics that once ingested will work around the clock to keep your gut in good shape. The experts are stressing more and more that so-called good gut bacteria is the key to good health. Having that said, yogurt is a safe way to get plenty of it. Yogurt certainly does help when it comes to your preparation for your intermittent fasting regimen.

Dark Chocolate

I know not everyone is a fan of dark chocolate, and perhaps it's an acquired taste. But whether it takes you a while to appreciate it or not, the health benefits are immediate. Dark chocolate gives you a boost of energy even while fortifying your system with valuable antioxidants. The kind of antioxidants capable of fighting off cancer no less. Simply put, dark chocolate is some powerful stuff. With so much going for it, dark chocolate is a go-to food when it comes to intermittent fasting.

Coconut Oil

Coconut oil is a low calorie, known metabolism booster, and will get your system up and running during your period of intermittent fasting. Coconut oil is good because it doesn't trigger insulin production unlike other oils do. You can use coconut oil as a supplement, or even a cooking aid, without any fear of disrupting your fast in the process. It's really quite a wonderful ingredient and you will see it made use of quite extensively in the recipes in this book.

What Not to Eat:

Soda

What no soda? You've got to be kidding me! Sorry, folks I like a good fountain drink of soda just like the next person, but I'm afraid it's all too true. If you want to engage in intermittent fasting, you are going to have to leave your soda behind. This is not meant as punishment—it's simply the reality of the beast. One of the major components of an intermittent fast after all, is the avoidance of sugar. It's so your body will start burning fat stores already in place that during fasting we refrain from guzzling sugary soda for our metabolic rate to nibble on. So yes, for the time being, as you engage in an intermittent fasting routine, you will indeed have to forego soda.

Heavily Processed Food

As you have probably already picked up on during the course of this book, processed foods are frowned upon. Anything that has been processed and packaged is going to have a ton of preservatives packed into them, that while generally harmless, will have a long-term effect on your system over time. Heavily processed food will also pose a direct interference with your metabolism. That's why the fresher the food, the better when it comes to intermittent fasting.

Sugary Sweets

Just like with sugary sodas, sugary sweets would be completely counterproductive for an intermittent fast. The goal of an intermittent fast after all is to switch the body from burning sugar and carbs, to burning our latent fat deposits instead. Eating sugary sweets would disrupt this process and instead just add more junk to the fat already deposited in our trunk. So yes, you must avoid sugary sweets at all cost while you participate in intermittent fasting.

Alcohol

I don't mean to be a party pooper or anything, but let me just go ahead and say it. Alcohol and intermittent fasting do not mix. The reason? Alcohol has a direct effect on fat burning metabolism. And the last thing that you would want to do is wreck your fast by throwing a wrench in your fat burning metabolism! Alcohol also carries, carbs, sugars, calories and the like. So, yeah just like drinking and driving—drinking and fasting should be avoided.

Refined Grains

Unlike whole grains, refined grains will indeed have a decidedly negative impact upon your fast. Refined grains once metabolized will actually turn directly into sugar. As already mentioned, a few times in this chapter, sugar will defeat the purpose of your fast. The whole purpose of intermittent fasting is to get your body to stop burning sugar as fuel and burn fat instead. Ingesting refined grains that turn into sugar therefore, completely negates this process. It will also raise your insulin levels. Having that said, refined grains are to be avoided if at all possible.

Trans-Fat

To be perfectly blunt, trans-fats are just bad. No good can come from them. And most especially, no good could come from your fast by ingesting them. Trans-fat, the fatty acids found in certain milk and meat products should be avoided while you participate in an intermittent fast. It raises, cholesterol, insulin, and wrecks any chance you may have had of having a successful fast. Just say no, when it comes to trans-fat.

Fast Food

Even though we call it "fast food"—the burgers and fries we bag from places like McDonald's are not exactly the best thing to eat during an intermittent fast! One look at an overly processed, carb dense meal from McDonald's and I think you might probably understand why.

At any rate, presented here are the foods that you should and shouldn't eat. Take note and take heart. Enjoy your fast!

Chapter 6:
Additional Tips and Tricks to Ensure a Successful Fast

Intermittent fasting doesn't have to be a struggle. In fact, if done right it can be quite enjoyable—even life changing. It's all just a matter of how you approach your fast. You've just got to do what you can to make the best of it. Having that said, here in this chapter we will go over some additional tips and tricks to get you on the right path and ensure that you have a successful fast.

Don't Get Bored

One of the biggest pitfalls of the intermittent fast is boredom. Mindless eating after all, often strikes simply because we don't have anything else to do. The more packed your itinerary is, the less likely you will succumb to eating out of sheer boredom. If you have a hobby, make full use of it. Blow off some steam with a pastime rather than mindlessly grazing through an afternoon. Just make sure that you don't get bored and you will be more likely to stay on track.

Satisfy Your Appetite with Zero Calorie Beverages

Simply drinking water or some other zero calorie beverage can help temporarily fill you up and satisfy your appetite while you fast. Water of course is a good and filling zero calorie beverage. It's nature's natural replenisher. But it's not the only one. Some good zero calorie beverages include:

- Coffee (Without cream or sugar)
- Spring Water
- Tea (Again, without cream or sugar)

Don't Get Overwhelmed

Many who start a regimen of intermittent fasting—especially if they have no previous experience with fasting—find themselves becoming a bit overwhelmed. Going into a fasting routine stressed out will only make things worse however, so whatever you do, make sure you don't stress out over your efforts. In order to avoid this, go into your intermittent fasting routine with the attitude that it's okay to make mistakes. If you slip up the first couple of times you fast, don't worry about it, just correct yourself and try again. Intermittent fasting after all—in many ways—is a trial and error process. You need to experiment and figure out exactly what works best for you, so be sure to give yourself enough breathing room to do so.

Have a Good Attitude

In many ways, this might seem like common sense, but it's worth saying regardless—attitude is everything. If you go into intermittent fasting with the attitude that you are going to fail, then it probably won't be long before you conclude a self-fulfilled prophecy. On the other hand, if you take on a good attitude of trying to be positive and make the best of things, you will be that much closer to success. It's really just as simple as that. And if you aren't in a good mood. Just fake it until you make it, and your spirits will begin to rise regardless.

Make Use of BCAAs

Just what are BCAAs you might ask? That fancy little acronym stands for "Branch Chain Amino Acids", and they are highly useful when it comes to girding your system for an intermittent fast. Among other things, BCAAs make sure that you do not lose too much muscle while your body is burning up all of that fat during a fast. And studies have shown that taking 10 g of a BCAA supplement before a fast can indeed really do some wonders.

Fast While you Sleep

Unless you are engaged in an intermittent fast that takes up a whole 24-hour period, it's always advisable to situate most of your fast time during your sleeping hours. This means you could usually simply skip dinner or breakfast, and then sleep off the rest of your fast. If for example, you want to fast for 16 hours, you could have an early evening meal at 5 PM and then not eat again until 9 AM the next morning. This would thereby complete a 16-hour fasting cycle without much feeling of deprivation involved. Just fast while you sleep and your body will do the rest.

Use Proper Portion Control

When it comes to successful intermittent fasting, being able to use proper portion control is crucial. If your fast day routine allows you to eat under 500 calories, portion control is of course necessary in order to keep yourself within your allotted limits. But perhaps even more importantly, should be the portion control you exercise when it comes to your non-fast days. For it is the non-fast day that will have you tempted to go overboard and eat too much if you are not careful.

Intermittent fasting after all, recommends someone to fast then eat normally, not fast and then binge! Because believe me, if someone starves themselves for 24 hours and then eats until they are absolutely stuffed the next day—they're not helping anyone! But there is a simple physiological reason that folks tend to get messed up when it comes to their portion control after a fast. You may notice that after the first few hours of a fast, you cease to feel hungry.

Hunger pains are the body's built in cue to eat. You may notice however, that after the first few hours of a fast, your hunger subsides. This is because by then our body realizes that food is not forthcoming. For the rest of your fast you may very well not feel all that hungry at all. But this is what happens folks. After you end your fast, and get out a bowl of pasta, the second you take that first bite, your body screams, "Oh wow—we have food now!"

And almost immediately the hunger pains hit you with abandon, and your body is now working you overtime to consume as much as you possibly can. It's just the way we are hardwired to be. Everything about the human condition is geared toward survival and our ancestors in the past went through periods of feast and famine—often not knowing when the next meal was going to be. So it is that our body's will turn off the hunger signal when we do without for a while, and yet will then poke, prod, and goad us into eating as much as possible when food is suddenly available.

That's great for someone who might not know when their next meal might be, but it's horrible for someone trying to plan a strategic intermittent fast under strict guidelines and protocol. That's why sometimes you might find yourself having to exercise a bit of mind over matter in order to keep yourself from overdoing it on your non-fast day and proper portion control can be a real lifesaver when it comes to intermittent fasting.

Closely Monitor Your Results

For most of us, nothing serves to encourage us more than seeing good, positive results. And as you fast, being able to monitor your progress will not only help you to improve problem areas, it will also give you a boost of self-confidence to show you how far you have come along in the process. Also, as intermittent fasting is in many ways a trial and error process, being able to track your journey in real-time enables you to tweak and finesse your experience until your methodology is at its most optimal. Everyone is different after all, and intermittent fasting isn't a one size fits all program. Having that said, monitoring your results will give you the feedback you need to make improvements when necessary, as well as provide you with solid encouragement as you go.

Chapter 7:
Make Your Shopping List and Plan Your Meals Accordingly

One of the most important things you can do when it comes to intermittent fasting is to make sure that you have proper supplies ahead of time and this means making a shopping list. But if your idea of shopping is buying heavily processed pre-packaged meals, you're going to have to make some adjustments. Because when it comes to being successful with intermittent fasting the fresher your food the better off you are going to be. The food you eat should also be well balanced, and taken from the following categories: Dairy, Fruits/Veggies, Spices, Nuts/Legumes, Meat, and Oil/Butter. In this chapter we will break it all down for you so that you know exactly what you should have on your shopping list so that you can then plan your meals accordingly.

Make Your Shopping List

Eggs/Dairy

Eggs and dairy are important building blocks for any fast, providing fortifying protein, calcium, and other nutrients. While beneficial however, they must be taken in moderation in order not to interfere with your fast. Also, when it comes to dairy, although you might think that it's a good idea to eat "low-fat dairy", this is simply not the case. Dairy has what we call "healthy fats" and they are a useful nutritional aid for your fast. In this instance you are actually going to want avoid the low-fat yogurt for example, since you need your dairy's natural fat to remain intact.

Cross these off your list:
- **Large Grade A Eggs**

Grade A eggs are the standard bearer, and these bad boys pack a protein punch and are useful for a wide variety of meals and recipes. If you really stop and think about it—it only makes sense that eggs are loaded with nutrition. Locked within the yolk of an egg after all is all the sustenance needed to grow a baby bird! Yes, it's true that gooey yellow egg-yolk is capable of growing a little chick! Now, just try to get that image out of your head as you sit down for scrambled eggs in the morning! At any rate, you can count on Large Grade A Eggs to come complete with vitamin A, vitamin B5, vitamin B12, Vitamin B2, and phosphorous, just to name a few vital nutrients.

- **Cottage Cheese**
Derived from curdled milk, cottage cheese is a good source of phosphorous, selenium, Vitamin B12, and protein. This combination of nutrients has a satiating effect on the body, helping to decrease appetite. Cottage cheese is good for you and good for your metabolism. You should always keep some in ready supply for your fast days.

- **Yogurt**
Yogurt is a dairy product similar to cottage cheese, except it is produced through the bacterial fermentation of milk. Yep, yogurt is the product of bacteria. It may not sound too appetizing to think that bacteria spawn's yogurt. But yogurt is in fact, an extremely nutritious food and the taste speaks for itself. It turns out that our little bacteria friends knew what they were doing, because yogurt is full of a little something called "probiotics." Eating yogurt can help you to maintain good gut bacteria that will in turn help you to make your intermittent fasting a stunning success.

- **Low-fat Shredded Cheese**
Cheese is of course, a staple of dairy food, and comes rich in abundance with calcium, protein, and phosphorus. But some cheeses are more fattening in

others. Having that said, it would do you good to find yourself a package of shredded cheese marked as low-fat. Standard, low-fat shredded cheese of all kinds can be made use of in a wide variety of intermittent fasting recipes. Whether you are sprucing up a scrambled egg melt, garnishing a cheesy casserole dish, or stuffing your tacos, low-fat shredded cheese is a vital ingredient. The next time you do some grocery shopping, be sure to add a good batch of low-fat shredded cheese to your cart.

- **Low-fat Buttermilk**
  Buttermilk is yet another dairy staple that is good for you and good in many meals and arrangements. It works as a stand-in and filler for many dishes but besides its culinary appeal, buttermilk has several great health benefits. Like yogurt, buttermilk provides a significant boost to the overall health of the body's gut. It is this microbial ecosystem in the digestive system that helps to not only digest nutrients, but also to locate, dismantle and discard harmful toxins. Buttermilk is yet another key to the puzzle when it comes to regulating this complicated piece of biological machinery. Be sure to add it to your shopping list.

Fruits/Veggies

Fruits and veggies should be a main staple as you progress through your intermittent fast. Many fruits such as bananas contain vital amounts of potassium, which is a proven safeguard against heart disease. Because potassium—among other things—helps us to ensure that our blood pressure stays low. Vegetables of course, have many crucial nutrients as well, such as iron. Did you know that iron exists in every cell of the body? Cellular function in fact depends upon, and it's for this reason that those who are anemic (low on iron) find themselves chronically fatigued. Needless to say, fruits and vegetables provide a great boon of nutrients that help us to be able to get through our day. And when it comes to fruit and vegetables—the fresher the better.

Here are a few items to consider for your shopping list:

- **Avocados**

    As tasty as it is, the avocado is quite healthy. The Avocado is yet another food that has "healthy fats." Rather than the trans fats that get you in trouble the fat found in avocado girds your body with strength, energy, and vitality. They also get rid of inflammation. So be sure and have some avocados on your shopping list.

- **Apples**

    You know what they say. An apple a day keeps the doctor away. It won't hurt your fast either! Apples are nutritious and loaded with antioxidants.

- **Carrots**

    Carrots aren't just for rabbits. They should also be a vital staple of your intermittent fasting routine.

- **Bananas**

    Bananas come loaded with not only potassium, but also fiber, and vitamin C. All of these nutrients serve as major regulators of bodily function. Potassium helps to regulate blood pressure, fiber regulates digestion, and vitamin C helps to reduce the incident of inflammation by keeping inflammatory molecules called free radicals in check. You'll find plenty of uses for bananas in this book, so don't neglect this vital resource.

- **Artichokes**

    Artichokes are a veggie to be reckoned with. These guys have their own set of valuable prebiotics to help improve your gut, as well as plenty of fiber to help you stay regular. These guys should be placed right at the top of your shopping list.

Spices

Spices can most certainly bring a little flair to an otherwise dull dish, but they do a lot more than that. Because just the right spice can actually help boost your metabolism and streamline your fast.

Here are a few to consider:
- **Cinnamon**
  Cinnamon actually has a phenomenal ability when it comes to the regulation of sugar in the blood. It is also loaded with antioxidants and can help reduce inflammation.
- **Turmeric**
  Ground from a root, a little bit of turmeric powder sprinkled on your food certainly goes a long way. Known to reduce inflammation and reinvigorate the body—turmeric can also aid in your intermittent fast.
- **Garlic powder**
  Garlic is a known immune booster, and it can also help boost your metabolism. Be sure to have some on hand.

Nuts/Legumes

Nuts and legumes are a low-calorie source of protein and as such they should be at the top of your grocery list when it comes to intermittent fasting. They are good for a snack, or as part of a main meal. Be sure to stock up on nuts and legumes.

Here are a few to consider for your list:
- **Almonds**
  Almonds are a powerful metabolism booster.
- **Lentils**
  Lentils are nutritious and full of protein.
- **Walnuts**
  Breakfast, dinner, or lunch—walnuts pack a punch!
- **Chick peas**

Chick peas are healthy for your fast and good for a wide variety of dishes.

Meat

While meat is important, when it comes to intermittent fasting; not all meats are created equal. Red meats should be avoided due to high fat contents, whereas lean chicken and fish should be a frequent offering during mealtime.

Add these meets to your shopping list:
- **Lean Chicken Breast**
  A piece of lean chicken breast is healthy, satisfying, and doesn't mess up your fast.
- **Salmon**
  Fish is said to be brain food and for good reason. Salmon can get you focused and ready for your fast. It's loaded with vitamin D and fortified with antioxidants.
- **Lamb**
  Lamb is well conducive for intermittent fasts.

Oils

This category is often neglected, but there are many valuable oils such as coconut and olive oil that can greatly aid the progress of your fast.

Oils to add:
- **Coconut Oil**
  Coconut oil boosts your metabolism and streamlines your fast.
- **Olive Oil**
  Olive oil is good for you, but be careful not to go over your calorie budget, because it packs significantly more calories than coconut oil does.

Now Plan Your Meals Accordingly

Here in this table you will find some suggested dishes based upon the shopping list of ingredients from the previous section. These dishes have been placed into various fasting regimens just to give you a basic idea of what to expect during an intermittent fasting routine. For the examples given below we are going to assume that the dieter is engaging in alternately timed, intermittent fasts starting on Monday, which includes under 500 calorie meals during their duration. Keep in mind that these are just suggestions to get you started however, and you are certainly free to mix and match meal plans, methods, and ingredients, as much as you would like.

For the 5:2 Method

Weekday	Breakfast	Lunch	Snack	Dinner	Dessert
Monday (fast)	Quiche Breakfast Dish	Lean Green Soup	Refreshing Green Smoothie	Salmon and Green Beans	Low Cal Cocoa
Tuesday	Cheesy Jalapeno Omelet	Sea Bass Fillets	Sunflower Cookies	Carrot Topped Pizza	Coconut Avocado Ice Cream
Wednesday (fast)	Refreshing Green Smoothie	Lean Beef Vegetable Soup	Low Cal Cocoa	Spicy Shrimp Stir fry	Peanut Butter Bars
Thursday	Indian Sweet Potatoes	Low Carb Cabbage Bowl	Chia Seed Pudding	Chicken Poblano Mix	Low Cal Lemon Curd
Friday	Poached Eggs Mushrooms and Tomatoes	Brown Rice Stir Fry	Homemade Dark Chocolate	Whole Wheat Spaghetti Dinner	Fasting Snickerdoodle Cookies
Saturday	Sweet Potato and Egg Casserole	Veggie Black Bean Burger	Sunflower Cookies	Moroccan Orange Chicken Meal	Chia Seed Pudding
Sunday	Spinach and Scrambled Eggs	Portobello Mushroom Fajita Wraps	Peanut Butter Bars	Chickpeas, Tomatoes, Broccoli, and Spinach	Sunflower Cookies

For the 12 Hour Fast

Weekday	Breakfast	Lunch	Snack	Dinner	Dessert
Monday	fast	Pineapple and Brown Rice	Low Cal Lemon Curd	Spicy Shrimp Stir Fry	fast
Tuesday	fast	Slow Cooked Spicy Chili	Peanut Butter Bars	Carrot Topped pizza	fast
Wednesday	fast	Sea Bass Fillets	Homemade Dark Chocolate	Beefy Maple Steak	fast
Thursday	fast	Lean Beef Vegetable Soup	Fasting Snickerdoodle Cookies	Chicken Vegetable Stew	fast
Friday	fast	Brown Rice Stir Fry	Low Cal Cocoa	Chicken Poblano Mix	fast
Saturday	fast	Portobello Mushroom Fajita Wraps	Sunflower Cookies	Moroccan Orange Chicken Meal	fast
Sunday	fast	Veggie Black Bean Burger	Chia Seed Pudding	Salmon and Green Beans	fast

For the 16 Hour Fast

Weekday	Breakfast	Lunch	Snack	Dinner	Dessert
Monday	fast	fast	fast	Portobello Mushroom Fajita Wraps	fast
Tuesday	fast	fast	fast	Carrot Topped Pizza	fast
Wednesday	fast	fast	fast	Tuna Fish Casserole Dish	fast
Thursday	fast	fast	fast	Beefy Maple Steak	fast
Friday	fast	fast	fast	Spicy Shrimp Stir Fry	fast
Saturday	fast	fast	fast	Moroccan Orange Chicken Meal	fast
Sunday	fast	fast	fast	Whole Wheat Spaghetti Dinner	fast

For the Weekly 24 Hour Fast

Weekday	Breakfast	Lunch	Snack	Dinner	Dessert
Monday	Cheesy Jalapeno Omelet	Lean Green Soup	Low Cal Lemon Curd	Whole Wheat Spaghetti Dinner	Chia Seed Pudding
Tuesday	Quiche Breakfast Dish	Brown Rice Stir Fry	Chia Seed Pudding	Portobello Mushroom Fajita Wraps	Fasting Snickerdoodle Cookies
Wednesday	Spinach and Scrambled Eggs	Pineapple and Brown Rice	Homemade Dark chocolate	Veggie Black Bean Burger	Coconut Avocado Ice Cream
Thursday	Indian Sweet Potatoes	Low Carb Cabbage Bowl	Peanut Butter Bars	Brown Rice Stir Fry	Low Cal Lemon Curd
Friday	Poached Eggs, Mushrooms, and Tomatoes	Seabass Fillets	Low Cal Cocoa	Carrot Topped Pizza	Sunflower Cookies
Saturday	Refreshing Green Smoothie	Lean Beef Vegetable Soup	Sunflower Cookies	Spicy Shrimp Stir Fry	Peanut Butter Bars
Sunday (24 fast)	MCT oil	glass of water	glass of water	glass of water	glass of water

Chapter 8:
Recipes of Suggested Dishes for Your Intermittent Fast

Now that we have gone over the basics of intermittent fasting, the methods, meal plans, and the like. Let's go ahead and delve right into some recipes and suggested dishes that will help you make the best of your intermittent fast. Here you will find a wide variety of foods and flavors to help you through your fast from sun up to sun down. Feel free to try them all.

Breakfast Recipes

Indian Sweet Potatoes

If you like Indian food, then you are going to love this 207-calorie dish! It comes complete with a batch of tasty sweet potatoes marinated with just the right mix of oil, lemon juice, and garlic. And the addition of nuts, cumin, and sesame seeds takes it to a whole other level. This dish makes for a relatively simple, yet absolutely perfect breakfast, lunch, or dinner for a fast day. You're going to love it!

Prep time: 10 minutes
Cook Time: 14 minutes
Total Time: 24 minutes

Per Serving
Calories: 207
Protein: 3 g
Carbs: 20 g
Fat: 14 g

Serves: 4

Ingredients:
- 1 tablespoon of olive oil
- 1 tablespoon of coconut oil
- 1 tsp of cumin seeds
- 1 tsp of sesame seeds
- 1 cup of chopped sweet potatoes
- ½ tsp of salt
- 2 tablespoons of chopped peanuts
- 1 tablespoon of lemon juice
- 1 tablespoon chopped garlic

Instructions:

1. Place a medium saucepan onto a burner set for high heat and add your tablespoon of olive oil.
2. Allow the oils to warm up a moment before adding your tsp of cumin seeds, followed by your tsp of sesame seeds.
3. Stir and cook your seeds in the pan for about 2 minutes.
4. Now add your cup of chopped sweet potatoes followed by your ½ tsp of salt, stir and cook for another 2 minutes.
5. Next, add your 2 tablespoons of chopped peanuts, followed by your tablespoon of lemon juice, and your tablespoon of chopped garlic, and stir it all together as it cooks for another 10 minutes.
6. Serve when ready.

Spinach and Scrambled Eggs

Healthy spinach blended into a tasty omelet—it's the recipe for a good morning!

Prep time: 8 minutes
Cook Time: 10 minutes
Total Time: 18 minutes

Per Serving
Calories: 235
Protein: 20 g
Carbs: 4 g
Fat: 228 g

Serves: 2

Ingredients:
- 1 cup of chopped spinach
- ¼ cup of diced onion
- 1 tablespoon of Frank's Hot Sauce
- ¼ tsp of salt
- ¼ tsp of pepper
- 2 tablespoons of olive oil
- 2 eggs

Instructions:
1. Place a medium sized saucepan onto a burner set for high heat and add your 2 tablespoons of olive oil to the pan.
2. Next, add your cup of shredded spinach and stir and cook it into the oil for about 1 minute, before transferring your spinach to a separate, medium sized bowl and set to the side.

3. Now add your ¼ cup of diced onion, and your tablespoon of Frank's Hot Sauce followed by your 2 eggs.
4. Vigorously stir the egg mixture, making sure the eggs do not stick to the pan, for about 2 minutes.
5. Once cooked, deposit the egg mixture into your bowl of spinach.
6. Season with your ¼ tsp of salt and your ¼ tsp of pepper and serve when ready.

Quiche Breakfast Dish

Do you like eggs loaded with just the right amount of onion, broccoli, and zucchini? Then checkout this Quiche Breakfast Dish! At just 124 calories this recipe comes loaded with all of the fixings. This tasty dish really gets your metabolism up running and ready for your fast. All in all—it's a great way to start your morning!

Prep time: 3 minutes
Cook Time: 20 minutes
Total Time: 23 minutes

Per Serving
Calories: 124
Protein: 9 g
Carbs: 2 g
Fat: 5 g

Serves: 4

Ingredients:
- 8 eggs
- 1 tsp of salt
- 1 tsp of pepper
- ½ cup of chopped onion

- ¼ cup of chopped zucchini
- ½ cup of chopped broccoli
- 2 tablespoons of olive oil

Instructions:

1. Set your oven for 350 degrees.
2. Now add your 2 tablespoons of olive oil to an oven safe dish and set to the side.
3. Get out a mixing bowl and add your 8 eggs, your tsp of salt, and your tsp of pepper.
4. Add your ½ cup of chopped onion, your ¼ cup of chopped zucchini, and your ½ cup of chopped broccoli to the bowl and stir everything together well.
5. Dump mixing bowl ingredients into your baking dish and cook for about 20 minutes.
6. Serve when ready.

Poached Eggs, Mushrooms, and Tomatoes

Tasty Poached Eggs, Mushrooms, and tomatoes—it doesn't get much better than that!

Prep time: 5 minutes
Cook Time: 15 minutes
Total Time: 20 minutes

Per Serving
Calories: 280
Protein: 17 g
Carbs: 5 g
Fat: 1 g

Serves: 2

Ingredients:
- 2 tsp of white vinegar
- 2 tablespoons of olive oil
- ¼ cup of diced tomatoes
- ½ cup of chopped mushrooms
- 1 tsp of shaved parmesan
- ¼ cup of water
- 4 eggs

Instructions:
1. To get started pour your ½ cup of water into a saucepan, followed by your 2 tablespoons of white vinegar and set your burner to medium heat.
2. While your saucepan heats up, place a frying pan onto a separate burner, set for high heat and add your 2 tablespoons of olive oil, your ¼ cup of diced tomatoes, and your ½ cup of chopped mushroom to the pan.
3. Stir and cook the ingredients together well over the next three minutes.
4. Next, break open each one of your eggs over a custard cup and place into the vinegar/water mixture in your saucepan. Cook for about 4 minutes under medium heat, before removing the poached eggs with a slotted spoon.
5. Arrange your poached eggs on a large plate or platter and serve with your cooked mushroom and tomato mixture.
6. Season with your tsp of shaved parmesan and serve when ready.

Cheesy Jalapeno Omelet

It tastes good and it's good for you! Get ready for a cheesy jalapeno blast! All you need are a couple of eggs, some garlic, jalapenos, and a bit of Monterey Jack and breakfast is served. If you need a little bit of spice in the morning, this dish gets the job done. And even loaded with cheese and jalapenos, this recipe is still able to keep you within your caloric budget during your fast!

Prep time: 2 minutes
Cook Time: 2 minutes
Total Time: 4 minutes

Per Serving
Calories: 187
Protein: 21 g
Carbs: 4 g
Fat: 8 g

Serves: 4

Ingredients:
- 2 eggs
- ½ cup of milk
- ¼ tsp of salt
- ¼ tsp of pepper
- 1 tablespoon of chopped garlic
- 1 tablespoon of chopped jalapeno pepper
- ½ cup of shredded Monterey Jack cheese

Instructions:
1. Get out a medium sized mixing bowl and add your 2 eggs, your ½ cup of milk, your ¼ tsp of salt, your ¼ tsp of pepper,

and your 1 tablespoon of chopped garlic, and mix everything together well.
2. Now place a large frying pan onto a burner set for high heat and deposit your mixing bowl ingredients inside.
3. Allow to cook for a minute or so, until the eggs become thick and lose their liquid consistency.
4. After this, deposit your tablespoon of chopped jalapeno pepper and your ½ cup of shredded Monterey jack cheese inside and use a spatula to carefully fold the egg over.
5. Cook for about another minute before turning the burner off.
6. This dish is ready to serve!

Sweet Potato and Egg Casserole

Casseroles comprise the ultimate comfort food. This dish makes use of 3 whole cups of cubed baked potatoes, tasty cheddar cheese, onions, and red bell pepper—and bacon. Yes, bacon! This is fasting dish designed to satisfy any lingering hunger pains you may have! Make it a part of your regular meal plan!

Prep time: 8 minutes
Cook Time: 40 minutes
Total Time: 48 minutes

Per Serving
Calories: 166
Protein: 10 g
Carbs: 7 g
Fat: 9 g

Serves: 1-2

Ingredients:
- 3 cups of cubed baked potatoes
- 6 eggs
- ¼ cup of sour cream
- ¼ tsp of salt
- 1 cup of milk
- ½ cup of shredded cheddar cheese
- 1 cup of chopped red bell pepper
- ½ cup of diced onion
- ¼ cup of olive oil
- ½ cup of chopped (already cooked) bacon

Instructions:
1. To get started, set your oven for 420 degrees, and evenly grease an oven safe cooking dish with your ¼ cup of olive oil. Deposit your 3 cups of cubed of baked potatoes into the dish and set to the side for the moment.
2. Now get out a large mixing bowl and add your 6 eggs, followed by your ¼ cup of sour cream, and your ¼ tsp of salt.
3. After this, add in your ½ cup of shredded cheddar cheese, your cup of chopped red bell pepper, your ½ cup of diced onion, and your ½ cup of chopped bacon, and mix everything together.
4. Dump mixing bowl ingredients over the potatoes and place the dish into the oven.
5. Cook for about 40 minutes.
6. Once cooked, allow to cool slightly, and serve when ready.

Lunch Recipes

Spicy Oven Baked Chicken

Lean chicken breast is a staple of intermittent fasting and this dish does not disappoint. Providing you with 2 lean chicken breasts slathered in buttermilk, whole wheat breadcrumbs and spicy brown mustard, it provides a unique and savory flavor.

Prep time: 10 minutes
Cook Time: 23 minutes
Total Time: 33 minutes

Per Serving
Calories: 248
Protein: 27 g
Carbs: 15 g
Fat: 2 g

Serves: 4

Ingredients:
- 4 tablespoons of fat-free buttermilk
- 2 tablespoons of spicy brown mustard
- 2 lean chicken breasts
- ¼ cup of whole wheat breadcrumbs
- ¼ cup chopped walnuts
- 1 tablespoon of chopped rosemary
- ¼ tsp of salt
- ½ tsp of pepper
- ½ tsp of cayenne pepper
- 2 tablespoons of honey

Instructions:
1. Set your oven for 425 degrees.
2. While your oven warms up, get out a medium sized mixing bowl and add your 4 tablespoons of fat-free buttermilk and your 2 tablespoons of spicy brown mustard.
3. Now place each chicken breast into the bowl, and turn them over in the mixture, until they are thoroughly coated.
4. Next, place a frying pan onto a burner set for high heat and add your ¼ cup of wheat breadcrumbs to the pan, followed by your ¼ cup of chopped walnuts, your 1 tablespoon of chopped rosemary, your ¼ tsp of salt, your ½ tsp of pepper, and your ½ tsp of cayenne pepper and stir everything together well as they cook over the next 2 to 3 minutes before turning the burner off.
5. Now place your buttermilk coated chicken into the pan and flip it around in the cooked breadcrumb ingredients until they are thoroughly coated with it as well.
6. Place your breadcrumb coated chicken breasts in an oven safe dish and cook for about 20 minutes.
7. Serve when ready.

Lean Green Soup

If you are looking for a midday meal that will help you recoup, just get a load of this bowl of Lean Green Soup! This soup comes complete with broccoli, parsley, and kale enhanced by the flavorings of garlic, turmeric, coriander, and coconut oil—cooked to perfection in a hearty batch of vegetable stock. Whether you are fasting or not, this Lean Green Soup hits the spot!

Prep time: 3 minutes

Cook Time: 9 minutes
Total Time: 12 minutes

Per Serving
Calories: 182
Protein: 10 g
Carbs: 14 g
Fat: 8 g

Serves: 4

Ingredients:
- 500 ml vegetable stock
- 1 tablespoon of coconut oil
- 1 tablespoon of minced garlic
- 2 tablespoons of water
- 1 tsp of coriander
- 1 tsp of turmeric
- ½ cup of chopped broccoli
- ½ cup of chopped kale
- ½ cup of chopped parsley

Instructions:
1. Add your tablespoon of coconut oil to a saucepan followed by your tablespoon of minced garlic, your tsp of coriander, and your tsp of turmeric.
2. Set the burner on high and add 2 tablespoons of water to the mix.
3. Stir ingredients together as they cook over the next 2 minutes.
4. Now add your 500 ml vegetable stock followed by your ½ cup of chopped broccoli, your ½ cup of chopped kale, and your ½ cup of chopped parsley.

5. Stir everything together well and allow to cook for another 7 minutes.
6. Allow to cool slightly, and serve when ready.

Portobello Mushroom Fajita Wraps

This dish boasts corn tortillas filled with delicious portobello mushrooms drenched in olive oil, garnished with onions, bell peppers, garlic, and jalapenos, with all the right seasonings applied. It's a feast that only consists of 207 calories. These portobello mushroom fajitas are wrapped up tight—and they will fill you up right!

Prep time: 10 minutes
Cook Time: 15 minutes
Total Time: 25 minutes

Per Serving
Calories: 207
Protein: 7 g
Carbs: 44 g
Fat: 2 g

Serves: 3

Ingredients:
- 3 corn tortillas
- 1 tablespoon of chopped jalapenos
- 2 tablespoons of olive oil
- 1 cup of chopped portobello mushrooms
- ¼ cup of chopped onions
- ¼ cup of chopped bell peppers
- 1 tablespoon of chopped garlic

- 1 tsp of cumin
- 1 tsp of smoked paprika
- ¼ tsp of salt

Instructions:

1. Get out a large pan and place it onto a burner set for high heat before adding your tablespoon of chopped jalapenos, your ¼ cup of chopped onions, your ¼ cup of chopped bell peppers, your tsp of cumin, your tsp of smoked paprika, and your tablespoon of chopped garlic.
2. Stir and cook all of your ingredients together for about 2 minutes.
3. After this, add your cup of chopped mushrooms.
4. Continue to stir and cook your ingredients over the next 10 minutes.
5. Evenly distribute your cooked ingredients into your tortillas and wrap them up.
6. This dish is ready to eat!

Brown Rice Stir Fry

What happens when you take a cup of brown rice, and dress it up nice with some broccoli, red bell pepper, zucchini, cabbage, and garlic? You have yourself one heck of a fast day meal at less than 200 calories a serving! Go ahead and give this Brown Rice Stir Fry a try!

Prep time: 2 minutes
Cook Time: 5 minutes
Total Time: 7 minutes

Per Serving
Calories: 197
Protein: 6 g

Carbs: 28 g
Fat: 8 g

Serves: 4

Ingredients:
- 1 cup of brown (cooked) rice
- 2 cups of chopped cabbage
- ½ cup of chopped broccoli
- ¼ cup of chopped red bell pepper
- ¼ cup of chopped zucchini
- 2 tablespoons of olive oil
- 1 tablespoon of chopped garlic
- 1 tablespoon of chopped parsley
- ¼ tsp of cayenne powder
- 1 tablespoon of soy sauce
- 1 tsp of sesame seeds
- 2 cups of water

Instructions:

1. To get started, add your 2 cups of water to a large frying pan followed by your 2 cups of chopped cabbage, your ½ cup of chopped broccoli, your ¼ cup of chopped red bell pepper, and your ¼ cup of chopped zucchini.
2. Set the burner on high and stir and cook over the next 3 minutes.
3. After this, drain any left-over water from the pan before setting it to the side.
4. Now place a wok (or similar cooking pan) onto a burner set for high heat and add your 2 tablespoons of olive oil, your tablespoon of chopped garlic, your tablespoon of chopped parsley, and cook for about 1 minute.

5. Next, add in your cooked vegetables followed by your cup of cooked rice, and stir and cook everything together for about a minute.
6. Drizzle your tablespoon of soy sauce, followed by your tsp of sesame seeds on top.
7. Serve when ready.

Low Carb Cabbage Bowl

It's low in carbs but high in taste. This Low Carb Cabbage Bowl provides a unique blend of carrots, onions, potatoes, and cabbage seasoned with turmeric and cumin. All ingredients offer up something very special in this eclectic culinary mix. You can rest assured that it's completely healthy—but it tastes so good!

Prep time: 3 minutes
Cook Time: 14 minutes
Total Time: 17 minutes

Per Serving
Calories: 327
Protein: 7 g
Carbs: 54 g
Fat: 18 g

Serves: 4

Ingredients:
- 2 tablespoons of olive oil
- ½ cup of chopped carrots
- ¼ cup of diced onions
- ½ tsp of salt
- ½ tsp of pepper
- 1 tsp of cumin

- ½ tsp of turmeric
- 1 cup of shredded cabbage
- 1 cup of chopped potatoes

Instructions:
1. Place a medium sized saucepan onto a burner set for high heat and add your 2 tablespoons of olive oil to the pan.
2. Next, add your ½ cup of chopped carrots, your ¼ cup of diced onions, your ½ tsp of salt, and your ½ tsp of pepper.
3. Stir and cook these ingredients for about 4 minutes before adding your cup of shredded cabbage, and your cup of chopped potatoes, followed by your tsp of cumin and your ½ tsp of turmeric.
4. Continue to stir and cook your ingredients for about 10 more minutes.
5. Turn the burner off, allow food to cool for a moment and serve.

Salmon and Green Beans

Salmon is good for cognition and focus, green beans meanwhile, are dense in iron and very nutritious. This recipe provides the perfect fuel for your fast, keeping the blood pumping and the mind in perfect concentration. Thanks to this Salmon and Green Beans, fish-based brain food has never been more delicious! Taking just 20 minutes of your time, this refreshing recipe is easy to make and even easier to eat!

Prep time: 3 minutes
Cook Time: 17 minutes
Total Time: 20 minutes

Per Serving
Calories: 330
Protein: 31 g
Carbs: 18 g
Fat: 12 g

Serves: 3

Ingredients:
- 1 tablespoon of chopped garlic
- 1 cup of chopped green beans
- 2 tablespoons of olive oil
- ½ tsp of salt
- ½ tsp of pepper
- 1 salmon fillet/sliced into 3 pieces
- 1 tablespoon of Greek yogurt

Instructions:
1. Preheat your oven to 425 degrees.

2. Now get out a greased baking sheet and add your tablespoon of chopped garlic, your cup of chopped green beans, and one of your tablespoon of olive oil, with your ½ tsp of pepper on top.
3. Place baking sheet into the oven and allow ingredients to cook for about 14 minutes.
4. After this, deposit your remaining tablespoon of olive oil into a medium sized frying pan, set the burner on high and add your 3 pieces of salmon fillet to the pan.
5. Sprinkle your ½ tsp of salt on top and cook the salmon fillet pieces for about 3 minutes on each side.
6. Once everything is cooked, add your fish to a plate alongside your baked green bean mix and it's ready to eat!

Carrot Topped Pizza

The chief complaint of many low-calorie diets is the loss of bread-heavy foods such as pizza. But don't worry folks! Because this recipe allows you to have your fast and eat your pizza too! Utilizing a non-refined, whole wheat pizza crust as a base, this pizza has a healthy dose of chicken, mozzarella cheese, and garlic, topped with carrots! And it only comes to 351 calories, so it can very well be squeaked into your fast day. If for example you are undergoing a 16 hour fast that allows you to eat one big caloric meal at the end of the day, this meal would do the trick. Check out this Carrot Toped Pizza for yourself!

Prep time: 5 minutes
Cook Time: 16 minutes
Total Time: 21 minutes

Per Serving
Calories: 351
Protein: 20 g
Carbs: 13 g
Fat: 11 g

Serves: 4

Ingredients:
- 2 tablespoons of rice vinegar
- 1 tablespoon of light brown sugar
- ½ cup of diced carrot
- ½ cup of water
- 1 tablespoon of olive oil
- 1 tsp of cornstarch
- 1 tablespoon of chopped garlic
- 1 cup of shredded (cooked) chicken
- 1 whole wheat pizza crust (already baked)

- ½ cup of mozzarella cheese

Instructions:
1. First, set your oven for 450 degrees.
2. Next, get out a mixing bowl and add your 2 tablespoons of rice vinegar, and your tablespoon of light brown sugar followed by your ½ cup of diced carrots.
3. Stir your carrots into the mixture until they are well coated.
4. Now get out an additional small mixing bowl and add your ½ cup of water followed by your tsp of cornstarch and briefly mix them together.
5. After this, place a small pan onto a burner set for high heat and add your tablespoon of olive oil followed by your tablespoon of chopped garlic.
6. Add your carrot mixture and your garlic mixture to the pan and stir everything together for about 4 minutes as it cooks.
7. Turn the burner off and add your cup of shredded (cooked) chicken, stir and cook over the residual heat for another 2 minutes.
8. Place your whole wheat pizza crust on a greased cooking sheet and evenly distribute your chicken mixture on top.
9. Sprinkle your ½ cup of mozzarella cheese over everything, place in oven, and cook for 10 minutes.
10. Your Carrot Topped Pizza is ready to eat!

Seabass Fillets

Are you a seafood fan? Well forget all about Red Lobster and try some of this seabass for your fast! At just 380 calories, this recipe makes use of 3 skinless seabass filets, tomatoes, spinach, olives, and cannellini beans, all garnished with just the right mix of garlic, salt, and pepper, cooked in a fine vegetable stock. This dish is good for lunch or dinner, on a fast or non-fast day alike. With these Sea Bass Fillets, there's a whole lot to like.

Prep time: 5 minutes
Cook Time: 9 minutes
Total Time: 14 minutes

Per Serving
Calories: 380
Protein: 40 g
Carbs: 15 g
Fat: 9 g

Serves: 3

Ingredients:
- 3 skinless seabass fillets
- ¼ tsp of salt
- ¼ tsp of pepper
- 2 tablespoons of olive oil
- 1 tablespoon of chopped garlic
- ½ cup of chopped tomatoes
- 1 cup of vegetable stock
- ½ cup of cannellini beans
- ½ cup of chopped baby spinach
- 1 tablespoon of lemon juice
- ½ cup of chopped olives

Instructions:
1. Get out a medium sized pan and place it on a burner set for high heat.
2. Add your 3 skinless seabass fillets followed by your ¼ tsp of salt, your ¼ tsp of pepper, your tablespoon of chopped garlic, and your 2 tablespoons of olive oil.
3. Stir fish into the pan as it cooks over the next 4 minutes.

4. Now add your ½ cup of chopped tomatoes, followed by your cup of vegetable stock, your ½ cup of cannellini beans, your ½ cup of chopped baby spinach, your tablespoon of lemon juice, and your ½ cup of chopped olives.
5. Continue to stir and cook your ingredients over the next 5 minutes.
6. Once cooked, turn the burner off and serve when ready.

Chicken Poblano Mix

If you are fasting and find yourself in need of a quick fix, then look no farther than this Chicken and Poblano Mix! This recipe takes a cup of shredded chicken and garnishes it with oregano, garlic, lime, and adobo sauce. This creates a potent flavor which the blunting effect of the poblano peppers do well to compliment. Poblano peppers work as a neutralizer and tend to take the bite out of more spicy components. This effect can be clearly seen in this recipe in the way that they interact with the adobo sauce. It is indeed a unique and eclectic mix, that works well to break up the monotony of your fast or non-fast days either one.

Prep time: 4 minutes
Cook Time: 17 minutes
Total Time: 21 minutes

Per Serving
Calories: 369
Protein: 20 g
Carbs: 44 g
Fat: 14 g

Serves: 2

Ingredients:
- 2 poblano peppers

- ¼ cup of olive oil
- 2 cups of diced onions
- 2 tablespoons of oregano
- 1 tablespoon of chopped garlic
- 1 cup of chopped tomato
- 2 tablespoons of adobo sauce
- ½ tsp of salt
- 1 tablespoon of lime juice
- 1 cup of (cooked) shredded chicken
- 2 cups of milk
- 1 cup of uncooked polenta

Instructions:
1. Get out a baking sheet and line it with aluminum foil.
2. Arrange your 2 poblano peppers to the sheet and drizzle your ¼ cup of olive oil over them.
3. Place in oven and broil for about 10 minutes.
4. Once cooked, chop the peppers into small pieces and set to the side.
5. Next, place a medium sized frying pan onto a burner ser for high heat.
6. Now add your 2 cups of diced onions, your 2 tablespoons of oregano, your tablespoon of chopped garlic, your cup of chopped tomato, your 2 tablespoons of adobo sauce, and your ½ tsp of salt.
7. Stir and cook your frying pan ingredients for about 5 minutes.
8. After this, add the cooked, chopped poblano peppers, your cup of cooked shredded chicken, and your tablespoon of lime juice to the pan and stir and cook everything for another 2 minutes.
9. Serve when ready.

Lean Beef Vegetable Soup

This soup features a hearty helping of lean ground beef, onions, tomato and cabbage. Portion control is key here, with the recommended serving size clocking in at just 160 calories. Eat it in a small bowl or a cup. If you feel like you're getting cold feet right in the middle of your fast, this bowl of Lean Beef Vegetable Soup will warm you right up! If you feel like you need a boost, give this recipe a try!

Prep time: 5 minutes
Cook Time: 25 minutes
Total Time: 30 minutes

Per Serving
Calories: 160
Protein: 14 g
Carbs: 12 g
Fat: 4 g

Serves: 2

Ingredients:
- 1 pound of lean ground beef
- 1 cup of chopped onions
- 3 cups of chopped cabbage
- 1 cup of diced tomatoes
- 1 pack of mixed vegetables
- ½ tsp of salt
- ½ tsp of pepper
- 1 cup of vegetable stock

Instructions:
1. Get out a medium sized frying pan and place it onto a burner set for high heat and add your pounds of lean ground beef to the pan.

2. Stir and cook the meat into the pan over the next 7 minutes.
3. Next, add your cup of chopped onions, followed by your 3 cups of cabbage, and your cup of diced tomatoes, and stir and cook everything together for another 5 minutes.
4. Once cooked, transfer ingredients to a large pot, pour in your 2 cups of vegetable stock, followed by your bag of mixed vegetables.
5. Set the burner on medium-high and stir and cook everything together for another 5 minutes.
6. Add your ½ tsp of salt and ½ tsp of pepper for flavor, and serve when ready.

Tuna Fish Casserole Dish

Need a good meal in a pinch? Then try this Tuna Fish Casserole Dish! Here you will find a whole cup of tasty tuna mixed with scrumptious elbow macaroni, and veggies, marinated in cream of mushroom soup and topped with minced carrots and pepper. So, if your fast is starting to make you fuss, just turn to this comfort food deluxe! It doesn't get much better than this!

Prep time: 5 minutes
Cook Time: 20 minutes
Total Time: 25 minutes

Per Serving
Calories: 227
Protein: 5 g
Carbs: 24 g
Fat: 8 g

Serves: 5

Ingredients:
- 2 cups (cooked) elbow macaroni

- ¼ cup of minced carrots
- 1 pack of mixed vegetables
- 1 cup of canned tuna
- ½ tsp of pepper
- 1 cup of canned cream of mushroom soup

Instructions:
1. Preheat your oven for 400 degrees.
2. Now get out an oven safe casserole dish and add you're your 2 cups of elbow macaroni, your ¼ cup of minced carrots, your pack of mixed vegetable, your cup of canned tuna, and your ½ tsp of pepper.
3. Next, pour your cup of canned cream of mushroom over the mix.
4. Put your casserole dish into the oven and cook for about 20 minutes.
5. Serve when ready.

Slow Cooked Spicy Chili

It's natural to get a bit fatigued when trying a fast. It takes our body some time to adjust. Having that said, a recipe like this works great to replenish much needed nutrients. This dish makes use of protein packed kidney beans for example, as well as iron rich spinach. Slow cooked to perfection, it's truly a fortifying mix of both sustenance and flavor. So, if you could use some self-sustaining protein for your fast, you don't have to go all willy-nilly. Just try something that really works—try some Slow Cooked Spicy Chili!

Prep time: 30 minutes
Cook Time: 5 hours
Total Time: 5 hours and 30 minutes

Per Serving
Calories: 134
Protein: 6 g
Carbs: 6 g
Fat: 25 g

Serves: 4

Ingredients:
- 2 tablespoons of olive oil
- ½ cup of chopped green bell pepper
- ½ cup of chopped red bell pepper
- ½ cup of chopped yellow bell pepper
- ¼ cup of chopped onion
- 1 tablespoon of chopped garlic
- 1 cup of chopped spinach
- 1 cup of corn
- ½ cup of chopped zucchini
- ½ cup of chopped yellow squash
- 5 tablespoons of chili powder
- 1 tablespoon of cumin
- 1 tablespoon of oregano
- 1 tsp of parsley
- ½ tsp of salt
- ½ tsp of pepper
- ½ cup of chopped tomatoes
- 1 cup of kidney beans
- 1 cup of chick peas
- ½ cup of tomato paste
- ½ cup of tomato sauce
- 1 cup of vegetable broth

Instructions:
1. To get started, place a medium sized frying pan onto a burner set for high heat and add your 2 tablespoons of olive oil to the pan.
2. Now add your ½ cup of green bell pepper, your ½ cup of red bell pepper, your ½ cup of tallow bell pepper, your ¼ cup of chopped onion, and your tablespoon of chopped garlic.
3. Stir and cook your ingredients over the course of the next 10 minutes.
4. After this, deposit the ingredients into a slow cooker, followed by your cup of chopped spinach, your cup of corn, your ½ cup of chopped zucchini, and your ½ cup of chopped yellow squash.
5. Now add your 5 tablespoons of chili powder, your tablespoon of cumin, your tablespoon of oregano, your tsp of parsley, your ½ tsp of salt, and your ½ tsp of pepper.
6. Briefly stir your ingredients and then add your ½ cup of chopped tomatoes, your cup of kidney beans, your cup of chick peas, your ½ cup of tomato paste, your ½ cup of tomato sauce, and your cup of vegetable broth.
7. Stir one more time before setting the cooker on high heat, placing the lid on top and allowing to cook for 5 hours.

Snacks/Dessert

Sunflower Cookies

At just 70 calories per serving, this tasty blend of sunflower seeds, turned cookies is a treat you won't forget. Cooked with coconut oil and baking soda, these cookies put your average chocolate chips to shame! If you need a great pick me up with no questions asked, these tasty sunflower cookies are just the dessert you need for your fast! So, the next time you are feeling hungry or overwhelmed, give this recipe a try!

Prep time: 2 minutes
Cook Time: 8 minutes
Total Time: 10 minutes

Per Serving
Calories: 70
Protein: 3 g
Carbs: 65 g
Fat: 6 g

Serves: 2
Ingredients:
- 1 egg
- ½ cup of sunflower seed butter
- 1 tablespoon of coconut oil
- 1 tablespoon of Truvia
- ½ tsp of vanilla extract
- ¼ tsp of baking powder
- ¼ tsp of baking soda
- ¼ tsp of salt

Instructions:
1. Set your oven for 360 degrees, and get out a slightly greased cookie sheet.
2. While your oven heats up, deposit your egg into your mixing bowl followed by your ½ cup of sunflower seed butter, your tablespoon of coconut oil, your tablespoon of Truvia, your ½ tsp of vanilla extract, your ¼ tsp of baking powder, your ¼ tsp of baking soda, and your ¼ tsp of salt.

3. Stir all of your ingredients together well before using your (clean) hands to form 8 individual clumps out of the mixture.
4. Arrange your clumps evenly on your greased cooking sheet and place the sheet into the oven.
5. Allow to cook for about 8 minutes or until golden brown.
6. Take out of oven and allow to cool.
7. Serve when ready.

Homemade Dark Chocolate

Dark chocolate is healthy and a proven superfood. And whether eaten as a snack or an after-dinner dessert, you should try to make it part of your fasting routine.

Prep time: 48 minutes
Cook Time: 0 minutes
Total Time: 48 minutes

Per Serving
Calories: 170
Protein: 2 g
Carbs: 15 g
Fat: 3 g

Serves: 2

Ingredients:
- 2 tablespoons of coconut oil
- ¼ cup of cocoa powder
- 2 tablespoons of honey
- 1 tsp of vanilla extract

Instructions:
1. Deposit your 2 tablespoons of coconut oil, followed by your ¼ cup of cocoa powder, your 2 tablespoons of honey, and your tsp of vanilla extract to a mixing bowl and spend a few minutes stirring it all together well.
2. Once thoroughly mixed together, cover the bowl and place it in the fridge for about 45 minutes.
3. Once chilled and hardened your Homemade Dark Chocolate is ready to eat!

Peanut Butter Bars

Here's a simple yet satisfying recipe which works well as both a snack in between meals, and as an after-dinner dessert.

Prep time: 6 minutes
Cook Time: 8 minutes
Total Time: 14 minutes

Per Serving
Calories: 116
Protein: 4 g
Carbs: 6 g
Fat: 5 g

Serves: 2

Ingredients:
- 1 cup of peanut butter
- ½ tsp of pure vanilla extract
- ¼ tsp of salt
- 2 tablespoons of almond flour
- ¼ cup of milk

Instructions:

1. Deposit your cup of peanut butter in to a mixing bowl, followed by your ½ tsp of pure vanilla extract, your ¼ tsp of salt, your 2 tablespoons of almond flour and your ¼ cup of milk.
2. Stir all of your ingredients together well and pour into an oven safe baking dish.
3. Place dish in oven and set temperature for 380 degrees.
4. Cook for about 8 minutes.
5. Take out of oven and allow to cool at room temperature.
6. Once cool, slice and serve.

Low Cal Lemon Curd

Low Cal Lemon Curd can't be beat! It's less than 100 calories on your plate, and it takes less than 10 minutes to make. With just three simple ingredients—an egg, lemon juice, and butter, this dessert is easy to make and even easier to eat!

Prep time: 4 minutes
Cook Time: 5 minutes
Total Time: 9 minutes

Per Serving
Calories: 74
Protein: 1 g
Carbs: 1 g
Fat: 7 g

Serves: 1-2

Ingredients:
- ¼ cup of lemon juice
- 1 egg
- ¼ cup of butter

Instructions:
1. Get out a small saucepan, place it onto a burner set for medium heat, and add your ¼ cup of butter.
2. Now add your egg and your ¼ cup of lemon juice and vigorously stir the mixture as it cooks together over the next 5 minutes.
3. Turn the burner off, transfer mixture to a dish and serve.

Coconut Avocado Ice Cream

If you like ice cream, then you are going to love this frost coconut avocado treat. As good as it tastes, it also comes complete with a tablespoon of MCT oil included, just to give you a little bit of an extra boost even as you treat yourself to a great tasting dessert. Just mix together your ingredients, chill in the fridge—and eat! At just 109 calories, this Coconut Avocado Ice Cream delivers in every way. Try it for yourself on your next fast day!

Prep time: 3 minutes and 4 hours
Cook Time: 0 (no cooking involved)
Total Time: 4 hours and 3 minutes

Per Serving
Calories: 109
Protein: 8 g
Carbs: 11 g
Fat: 90 g

Serves: 2

Ingredients:
- 1 large avocado
- 1 cup of coconut milk
- 1 tablespoon of MCT oil
- 1 tablespoon of lemon juice
- 1 tsp of minced mint leaves
- ¼ tsp of salt

Instructions:
1. First off, remove the pit and skin from your avocado, before placing your avocado, along with your cup of coconut milk,

your tablespoon of MCT oil, your tablespoon of lemon juice, and your tsp of minced mint leaves into a blender and blend for about 1 minute.
2. Now pour mixture into a plastic bowl and place into your freezer.
3. Freeze for about 4 hours before eating.
4. Serve when ready.

Fasting Snickerdoodle Cookies

I used to love snickerdoodles when I was a kid, and this recipe doesn't disappoint. It's a blast from the nostalgic past. It tastes just as good as any other traditional snickerdoodle recipe except without all those pesky carbs and calories. So, if you enjoyed these guys as much as I did back in the day, you are going to want to give this recipe a try.

Prep time: 3 minutes
Cook Time: 8 minutes
Total Time: 11 minutes

Per Serving
Calories: 105
Protein: 5 g
Carbs: 3 g
Fat: 25 g

Serves: 4

Ingredients:
- 1 cup of butter
- ½ cup of almond flour

- ½ cup of coconut flour
- 1 egg
- ¼ cup of baking powder
- 1 tablespoon of baking soda
- 1 tsp of cinnamon

Instructions:
1. To get started, preheat your oven for 350 degrees.
2. Now get out a medium sized mixing bowl and add your cup of butter, followed by your ½ cup of almond flour, your ½ cup of coconut flour, your egg, your ¼ cup of baking powder, your tablespoon of baking soda, and your tsp of cinnamon.
3. Stir all of your mixing bowl ingredients together well before using your (clean) hands to form them into 8 individual clumps.
4. Arrange your cookie clumps onto a greased baking sheet and place into the oven.
5. Allow to cook for about 8 minutes or until golden brown.
6. Let cookies cool and serve when ready.

Chia Seed Pudding

It's a refreshing treat made of coconut milk, cinnamon, and chia seeds. From one fast day to the next, this dessert keeps you on a solid footing. A tasty dessert that won't break your fast! Go ahead and try this Chia Seed Pudding! You'll be glad you did!

Prep time: 3 minutes and 3 hours
Cook Time: 0 minutes (No cooking involved)
Total Time: 3 hours and 3 minutes

Per Serving
Calories: 95
Protein: 2 g
Carbs: 2 g
Fat: 10 g

Serves: 1-2

Ingredients:
- ½ cup of coconut milk
- ¼ cup of chia seeds
- 1 tablespoon of Truvia
- 1 tsp of cinnamon
- ¼ tsp of salt

Instructions:
1. First, take your ½ cup of coconut milk, followed by your ¼ cup of chia seeds, your tablespoon of Truvia, your tsp of cinnamon, your ¼ tsp of salt, and your ¼ tsp of cinnamon and deposit them into a mixing bowl.
2. Now stir all of your ingredients together thoroughly for a couple of minutes.
3. Once mixed together, place plastic over the bowl and place it in the fridge.
4. Allow the mix to chill in the fridge for about 3 hours and serve when ready.

Refreshing Green Smoothie

Fasting is a commitment and it has its ups and it has its downs. But no matter where you may be on your fasting journey, this Refreshing Green Smoothie will rejuvenate your efforts. This green smoothie is ideal for breakfast or lunch during a fast day.

Prep time: 8 minutes
Cook Time: 9 minutes
Total Time: 17 minutes

Per Serving
Calories: 202
Protein: 2 g
Carbs: 4 g
Fat: 0 g

Serves: 2

Ingredients:
- 1 cup of apple juice
- ½ cup of chopped apple
- ½ cup of sliced avocado

Instructions:
1. Get out a blender and deposit your cup of apple juice followed by your ½ cup of chopped apple, and your ½ cup of sliced avocado.
2. Now simply hit the blend button and thoroughly blend everything together for a couple of minutes.
3. After this, just pour the mix right into a glass, drink up, and enjoy!

Low Cal Cocoa

If you're feeling a bit down in the dumps, this tasty cup of hot cocoa will help keep you alert! It's good as a quick breakfast, snack or dessert!

Prep time: 3 minutes
Cook Time: 1 minutes
Total Time: 4 minutes

Per Serving
Calories: 22
Protein: 1 g
Carbs: 3 g
Fat: 0 g

Serves: 1-2

Ingredients:
- 1 tablespoon of unsweetened cocoa powder
- 2 tablespoons of Splenda
- ¼ tsp of vanilla extract
- 1 cup of hot water

Instructions:
1. Add a cup of water to a coffee mug and heat up in the microwave for about 2 minutes.
2. Now deposit your tablespoon of unsweetened cocoa powder into a coffee mug, followed by your 2 tablespoons of Splenda, and your ¼ tsp of vanilla extract and stir it all together well.
3. Allow to cool slightly, and enjoy!

Dinner Recipes

Pineapple and Brown Rice

This dish had me at pineapple! Yes, this is another recipe with brown rice. Who says you can't have a good thing twice? With two servings, you can either share it, save some for later, or have a second helping. Either way you slice it, this Pineapple and Brown Rice dish is second to none. Feel free to serve this one up for lunch or dinner on a fast or non-fast day either one.

Prep time: 4 minutes
Cook Time: 7 minutes
Total Time: 11 minutes

Per Serving
Calories: 231
Protein: 9 g
Carbs: 22 g
Fat: 1 g

Serves: 2

Ingredients:
- ½ cup of chopped carrots
- 1 cup of chopped pineapple
- ½ tablespoon of soy sauce
- ½ tablespoon of Worcestershire sauce
- 1 cup of chicken broth
- ¼ tsp of salt
- 1 cup of (cooked) brown rice
- ½ cup of diced onions

Instructions:
1. Place a medium sized frying pan onto a burner set for high heat and add your ½ cup of chopped carrots, followed by your cup of chopped pineapple to the pan.
2. Next add your ½ tablespoon of soy sauce, your ½ tablespoon of Worcestershire sauce, your cup of chicken broth and your ¼ tsp of salt.
3. Stir and cook ingredients for about 5 minutes.
4. Now add your cup of cooked brown rice and your ½ cup of diced onions, stir and cook everything for another 2 minutes.
5. Serve when ready.

Chicken Vegetable Stew

Are you feeling a little weary? Like you're about to call it quits right in the middle of your fast? Don't worry, such things are understandable. That's why in order to get around it you need to have good recipes to hold you over during your fast days. At just 270 calories, this Chicken Vegetable Stew recipe provides a refreshing blend of lean chicken breast, veggies, and just the right amount of seasoning. So if you find yourself feeling a little blue—just eat your Chicken Vegetable Stew!

Prep time: 3 minutes
Cook Time: 20 minutes
Total Time: 23 minutes

Per Serving
Calories: 270
Protein: 2 g
Carbs: 2 g
Fat: 10 g

Serves: 1-2

Ingredients:
- ½ tablespoon of olive oil
- 1 cup of chopped chicken breast
- ¼ tsp of salt
- 1 cup of chopped potatoes
- 2 cups of vegetable stock
- 1 tablespoon of corn starch
- 1 tablespoon of water
- 1 cup of mixed vegetables
- ¼ tsp of salt
- ¼ tsp of pepper

Instructions:
1. Deposit your ½ tablespoon of olive oil into a medium sized pan and set your burner on high.
2. Now add your cup of chopped chicken breast, followed by your ¼ tsp of salt.
3. Stir everything together for about 5 minutes as it cooks.
4. Next add your cup of chicken broth, followed by your cup of chopped potatoes, your cup of mixed vegetables, your ¼ tsp of salt, and your ¼ tsp of pepper and cook for another 5 minutes.
5. Allow to cool slightly and serve whenever you are ready.

Spicy Shrimp Stir Fry

Fasting can be a daunting process. This dish provides a refreshing means of sustenance during the hardship. Loaded with shrimp, asparagus, and seasoned with cayenne pepper, on a fast day, this Spicy Shrimp Stir Fry, is sure to catch your eye!

Prep time: 3 minutes
Cook Time: 15 minutes
Total Time: 18 minutes

Per Serving
Calories: 235
Protein: 23 g
Carbs: 8 g
Fat: 12 g

Serves: 3

Ingredients:
- ¼ cup of olive oil
- 2 cups of shrimp
- 1 cup of chopped asparagus
- ¼ tsp of salt
- ¼ tsp of cayenne pepper

Instructions:
1. Place a medium sized frying pan onto a burner set for high heat and deposit your ¼ cup of olive oil into the pan.
2. Now add your 2 cups of shrimp to the pan, followed by your ½ tsp of salt, and your ¼ tsp of cayenne pepper.
3. Stir and cook for about 2 minutes before adding your cup of chopped asparagus to the pan.
4. Now stir and cook for another 5 minutes.
5. Serve when ready.

Chickpeas, Tomatoes, Broccoli, and Spinach

This meal is simple but delicious and brings together three staple foods of any fast—Chickpeas, Tomatoes, Broccoli, and Spinach. This dish makes for a great lunch or dinner. And at only 295 calories per serving, this recipe works for both fast and non-fast days.

Prep time: 5 minutes
Cook Time: 25 minutes
Total Time: 30 minutes

Per Serving
Calories: 295
Protein: 14 g
Carbs: 45 g
Fat: 8 g

Serves: 4

Ingredients:
- 1 cup of chopped onions
- 1 tablespoon of minced garlic
- 2 tsp of coriander
- ½ tsp of cumin
- ½ tsp of turmeric
- 1 tsp of chili powder
- ¼ tsp of salt
- 1 cup of chopped tomatoes
- 1 cup of chopped broccoli
- 2 cups of chickpeas
- 1 cup of chopped spinach
- 2 tablespoons of olive oil

Instructions:
1. Get out a large frying pan and place it onto a burner set for medium heat.
2. Deposit your 2 tablespoons of olive oil into the pan, followed by your cup of chopped onions and tablespoon of minced garlic.
3. Stir and cook your ingredients for about 4 minutes.
4. Now add your 2 tsp of coriander, your ½ tsp of turmeric, your ½ tsp of cumin, your tsp of chili powder, and your ¼ tsp of salt.
5. Stir everything together and cook for another 2 minutes.
6. Finally, add your cup of chopped broccoli, your 2 cups of chopped spinach, and your cup of chopped tomatoes into the pan.
7. Stir and cook everything together for another 5 minutes.
8. Serve whenever you are ready to do so.

Whole Wheat Spaghetti Dinner

Pasta is the bane of many dieters. Traditional pasta after all is one of the most carbohydrate dense foods you could ever eat. It's for this reason that runners often load up on linguine, lasagna, and spaghetti before a marathon, it's because they need plenty of carbs to burn for their run. But unless you are ready to run miles and miles, for most of us, such carb dense foods are simply not a good option. So, what is a pasta lover to do? Just switch from refined grain pasta to unrefined whole wheat and you will be fine. Yes, it's true. And this dish is exemplary of that fact. If you love pasta, you are really going to love this Whole Wheat Spaghetti Dinner.

Prep time: 5 minutes
Cook Time: 12 minutes
Total Time: 17 minutes

Per Serving

Calories: 395
Protein: 16 g
Carbs: 32 g
Fat: 11 g

Serves: 2

Ingredients:
- 7 ounces of (already cooked) whole wheat spaghetti
- 2 tablespoons of olive oil
- 3 ounces of turkey sausage
- 1 cup of diced onion
- 1 tablespoon of minced garlic
- ½ cup of chopped shitake mushrooms
- ½ cup of chopped yellow bell pepper
- ½ cup of tomato paste
- 1 cup of chopped broccoli
- ¼ tsp of salt
- ¼ tsp of cayenne pepper
- ½ cup of diced tomatoes

Instructions:
1. Inside a medium saucepan, on a burner set on high, add your 2 tablespoons of olive oil, followed by your 3 ounces of turkey sausage.
2. Vigorously stir the turkey sausage into the oil as it cooks over the course of the next 5 minutes.
3. Next, add your cup of diced onion, and tablespoon of minced garlic, and stir and cook for another 2 minutes.
4. Follow this by adding your ½ cup of chopped shitake mushrooms, and your ½ cup of chopped yellow bell pepper.
5. Cook and stir for another 3 minutes before adding your ½ cup of tomato paste.

6. Now add your cup of chopped broccoli, your ¼ tsp of salt, your ¼ tsp of cayenne pepper, and your ½ cup of diced tomatoes.
7. Reduce your burner to low heat and stir and cook everything together for another 2 minutes. Once cooked, this mix constitutes what will make up your spaghetti sauce.
8. Finally, add your already cooked whole wheat spaghetti to a plate and pour as much of your cooked spaghetti sauce ingredients on top.
9. Enjoy!

Moroccan Orange Chicken Meal

For a dinnertime dish with more than a little flare, try this Moroccan Chicken Meal. It comes fully equipped to deliver tasty chicken, veggies, and walnuts to your taste buds. Having that said, it is a little bit heavier on the calories, so it might work better as the one big meal you might use to break your fast after a 12-hour or 16-hour stint of not eating. At any rate, try this recipe out for yourself! You won't be disappointed!

Prep time: 8 minutes
Cook Time: 9 minutes
Total Time: 17 minutes

Per Serving
Calories: 422
Protein: 45 g
Carbs: 32 g
Fat: 11 g

Serves: 2

Ingredients:

- 2 lean chicken breasts
- ¼ tsp salt
- ¼ tsp pepper
- ¼ cup of olive oil
- 1 cup of chopped cauliflower
- ½ cup of chopped carrots
- ½ cup of diced onion
- 1 tablespoon of orange juice
- ¼ cup of walnuts

Instructions:
1. Lay out your 2 lean chicken breasts onto a clean, flat surface.
2. Now, take out a rolling pin and use it to flatten the chicken breasts as much as possible.
3. Once flattened season the chicken with your ¼ tsp of salt and your ¼ tsp of pepper.
4. Next, place a pan onto a burner set for medium heat and deposit your ¼ cup of olive oil into the pan.
5. Wait about a minute for the oil to warm up before placing your seasoned chicken into the pan.
6. Now cook your chicken breasts for about 3 minutes on each side.
7. After this, reduce the burner's temperature to low heat and add your ½ cup of chopped carrots, your cup of chopped cauliflower, and your ½ cup of diced onions to the pan.
8. After this add your tablespoon of orange juice on top, and cook and stir your ingredients together for another 5 minutes
9. Finally, top the ingredients off with your ½ cup of walnuts and serve when ready.

Veggie Black Bean Burger

If you find yourself missing burgers and fries during your fast, we've won half the battle for you right here. Because this Veggie Black Bean Burger tastes so much like an authentic hamburger that you won't even know the difference. Go ahead and try one for yourself today!

Prep time: 8 minutes
Cook Time: 9 minutes
Total Time: 17 minutes

Per Serving
Calories: 422
Protein: 45 g
Carbs: 32 g
Fat: 11 g

Serves: 3

Ingredients:
- ½ cup of chopped sweet potatoes
- 2 tablespoons of dry millet
- ¼ cup of rolled oats
- 1 tablespoon of cilantro
- 1 tablespoon of minced garlic
- 2 tsp of cumin
- ¼ tsp of salt
- 1 tsp of pepper
- 2 cups of black beans
- 1 and ½ cups of corn
- ¼ cup of olive oil
- 6 whole wheat hamburger buns

Instructions:
1. For starters, set your oven for 420 degrees.
2. After your oven warms up, get out a baking dish, put your ½ cup of chopped sweet potatoes inside and cook them for about 30 minutes.
3. Once cooked, transfer the cooked sweet potatoes to a blender, followed by your 2 tablespoons of dry millet, your ¼ cup of rolled oats, your tablespoon of cilantro, your tablespoon of minced garlic, your 2 tsp of cumin, your 2 cups of black beans, and your 1 and a ½ cups of corn.
4. Hit the blend button and allow to blend together for about 2 minutes.
5. Next, place a large frying pan onto a burner set for high heat and add your ¼ cup of olive oil to the pan.
6. Now deposit large clumps of your blended ingredients into the pan.
7. Once your clumps of blended ingredients are in place, get out a spatula and use it to flatten the clumps as they cook under the heat.
8. Cook burgers on both sides for about 3 minutes, flipping them over with your spatula.
9. Season with your ¼ tsp of salt and your tsp of pepper, and serve up each patty between a whole wheat hamburger bun.

Beefy Maple Steak

This dish really does use an eclectic mix of seasoning and it pays off well. Savory steak soaked in maple syrup and offset by the tangy flavor or Worcestershire and soy sauce. This great tasting meal comes to just over 200 calories and can be cooked up in about 15 minutes. It fits right in with your busy schedule whether it's a fast day or not. So, don't you hesitate. Go ahead and make your Beefy Maple Steak!

Prep time: 5 minutes

Cook Time: 10 minutes
Total Time: 15 minutes

Per Serving
Calories: 205
Protein: 2 g
Carbs: 4 g
Fat: 0 g

Serves: 2

Ingredients:
- ½ pound of sirloin steak
- 3 tablespoons of cornstarch
- 2 tablespoons of olive oil
- ¼ cup of beef broth
- 1 tablespoon of soy sauce
- ½ tablespoon of Worcestershire sauce
- 1 tablespoon of maple syrup
- 1 tablespoon of chopped garlic
- ½ tsp of cayenne pepper

Instructions:
1. Place a large frying pan onto a burner set on high and ad your ½ pound of sirloin steak and 2 tablespoons of cornstarch, and 2 tablespoons of olive oil.
2. Now cook the steak for about 3 minutes, thoroughly cooking each side.
3. Next, get out a small mixing bowl and add your ¼ cup of beef brother, your tablespoon of soy sauce, your ½ tablespoon of Worcestershire sauce, your tablespoon of maple syrup, your tablespoon of chopped garlic, and your ½ tsp of cayenne pepper.

4. Stir all of these ingredients together well before pouring them directly onto your cooked steak.
5. Your Beefy Maple Steak is ready to serve!

Chapter 9:
The Recipe for Success: Balanced Diet, Sleep, and Adequate Exercise

When it comes to your health, having a balanced diet, a good amount of sleep and adequate exercise is everything. And this doesn't change just because you are engaged in an intermittent fast. These three facets of life are crucial—there's no way around it. Just because you are fasting doesn't mean you can neglect either one of these pillars of health. Having that said, you just might wonder what the best approach toward diet, sleep and exercise might be. We'll go over them now.

Having a Balanced Diet

Yes, even while engaged in an intermittent fast, you must make sure that the foods that you do eat, are properly balanced. This means getting enough fruits, veggies, dairy, and meat to make sure that none of those major food groups are neglected. With your body able to take advantage of nutrients from a balanced diet, your system will be better able to withstand the rigors of a fast while burning off fat. Having the right amount of protein in your system for example will ensure that you do not lose muscle mass, while having enough calcium will prevent your bones from becoming depleted.

These two examples are rather obvious, but there are also some not so obvious examples as to why a well-balanced diet with plenty of vitamins and minerals will give you an edge. Because a well-balanced diet will boost not only your metabolism but your immune system, better enabling you to fight off illness. Your intermittent fasting routine after all, is not going to do you very much good if you come down with a cold or the flu! Eating the right kinds of food will also invariably give you more energy and even improve your mood—all of which will make your fasting routine, all the more successful in the end.

Getting the Right Amount of Sleep

You need sleep. This of course should be a no-brainer, but for many of us in this busy world, being able to get enough shuteye could very well seem much easier said than done. Many of us have schedules that have us frequently working long hours in the evening and yet still waking up early in the morning. But in the long run, such a routine is just not sustainable.

Not only that. It really tends to wreck our hormones. Because as we build up a deficit in sleep our body begins to release stress hormones such as cortisol, as well as insulin, which both contribute to weight gain. You could try to restrict even more calories, or do more exercise to counteract it, but it's a losing battle. So instead of struggling just make sure you get the right amount of sleep each night (or day, for you night owls), which for most adults would be at least 7 hours. Now that's not saying that the occasional night of getting just 5 hours of sleep will completely wreck your routine, but just don't make it a habit.

Achieving the optimal level of sleep will benefit every aspect of your day. You will have more energy of course, and your own physiology will be more conducive to both your fast and any exercise you might engage in. You also won't be ravenously hungry! Because lack of sleep will most certainly play havoc on your appetite. At any rate, the moral of the story here folks is—get the right amount of sleep!

Achieving Adequate Exercise

Yet many may wonder if it's safe to exercise during an intermittent fast. With the body depleted of nutrients during a fast after all, would it be wise to put it through any more strain than it's already under? According to the data, exercise while undergoing a fast has a direct effect on metabolism and the body's level of insulin. Both are activated with one going up and the other going down as the body recalibrates and begins to burn fat rather than carbs.

Engaging in the right kind of workout will help to speed up this process even more. Having that said, here are some exercises to give your intermittent fast a major boost.

- **Running/Treadmill**
  There is really nothing better to get the body's metabolic cylinders running than a good run. As soon as your feet hit the pavement (or the treadmill), your heart rate increases and the blood starts to much more vigorously pump through your body. With your bodily processes instantly speeding up like this, it's really no wonder that your metabolism might speed up as well. And this is precisely the case when you engage in this type of exercise during a fast. But having that said, just keep in mind that you have to be careful not to overdo it. And in order to ensure that you have the best experience, it is recommended that you only run during the first few hours of your fast. That way your body still has plenty of additional resources left over from the last meal you had before your fast began. If for example you began your fast at 10 PM on a Thursday night, you should be good to run around the block at 7AM Friday morning without any trouble. It is not advisable however to overexert yourself at the very end of your fast. Although most could probably handle it, just to be on the safe side, you should keep your running hours locked into the first few hours of your fast. Every step you take causes hormones to alert your metabolic engines that you are up and quite literally *running*.

- **Weight Lifting**
  If you are a weight lifter, or interested in becoming one—I have some good news for you. Lifting weights does not interfere with your fast! In fact, lifting weights during a fast can prove quite beneficial. As mentioned previously in this book, the very style of intermittent fasting is

designed to prevent muscle loss during fasting periods, but having that said, a little weight lifting will help to shield your body from muscle loss even more. Because the truth is, we all lose muscle as we age and if we don't work at maintaining it through muscle lifting, we just might find that our muscle mass declining significantly through the years. Even more beneficial for those wishing to lose weight, lifting weights during an intermittent fast also quickens the pace of fat burn even more. Just think about it, during a fast your body has already switched to burning fat for its fuel, so when you grunt, struggle, and strain to lift those weights, guess what your body's tapping into for energy? All that fat you want to get rid of! Do I dare say—this is a win win situation? It most certainly is!

- **Pushups**
  One of the most traditional exercises you could ever even consider would be that of the classic pushup. Pushups have been around forever and there is a reason for that—they are highly effective. By making use of gravity and your own body weight, the push up gets the heart going while the muscles do overtime to push the body up off the floor by virtue of arm strength alone. These exercises if done moderately—say no more than 20 to 30 pushups during a fast—can be highly effective in boosting your metabolism to the max, allowing an even more rapid depletion of the body's fat stores. This is some good news that you could most certainly use!

- **Squats**
  This is another great exercise that seems absolutely made for intermittent fasting. Squats focus on your glutes, quads and other muscles like there is no tomorrow! This exercise keeps you going and keeps you strong! As you might imagine, squats consist of the participant bending

their knees and squatting down toward the ground as if they are sitting on a chair. This bending motion gets the blood flowing to the thighs and begins rapidly burning fat deposits. If you need to target fat in the legs in particular, you might want to give this exercise a try.

- **Dips**
  Why yes—we would be remiss if we did not mention dips! And no, I'm not talking about the stuff you dip your chips in at the football game, I'm talking about high intensity, fat busing exercise that will burn fat, boost your metabolism and make sure your upper body stays nice and strong. These exercises are just about perfect for intermittent fasting as they get the blood flowing without making you too tired in the process.

- **Planks**
  Planks are a fairly common yet highly efficient exercise that can be done at home, at the gym, or just about any place you may be at the time. This exercise is also quite nuanced and flexible when it comes to adjusting the intensity and the area of focus. Planks tend to build up quite a bit of endurance too, which is most certainly good for someone who is undergoing a fast. It is best to engage in this exercise during the first few hours of your fast, but they can be done periodically throughout the rest of the fasting day as well.

- **Reverse Lunge**
  This exercise may look easy at first glance but don't be fooled. Reverse lunges are a high intensity workout that gets your metabolism going. And when done during a fast, it really kicks things into high gear. They are also good for getting your legs in tip top shape which is beneficial for just about every other aerobic exercise you could do.

- **Burpee**
    No, a burpee isn't what happens when you eat too many hot peppers. A bad joke maybe, but in all seriousness, there are many out there who are confused with what a burpee is and what it is not. The Burpee is a classic hybrid styled exercise that makes full use of cardio as well as resistance exercises, in order to maximize your metabolism. These exercises are pretty intensive, so if you are engaged in a less than 500 calorie fast day, you might want to actually have a low-calorie snack or other healthy option. Good choices for nutrition before this workout would be perhaps just a 1 hard-boiled egg, a salad, or maybe even a bowl of chicken broth. Either way, these workouts are sure to get your body running on all cylinders during your intermittent fast.

As you can see, the benefits of a well-balanced diet, sleep, and exercise cannot be stressed enough. No matter what kind of fasting regimen you decide upon, you need to make sure that these rudimentary needs are taken care. Burning fat and losing weight after all, should be treated from a holistic standpoint, in which the overall health and wellbeing of the body is taken into consideration. Regardless of anything else, this indeed is the true recipe for success.

Chapter 10:
Some Intermittent Fast FAQs

As you start off on an intermittent fast, you probably have a lot of questions. Hopefully, many of them have already been answered for you during the course of reading this book. Just in case however, let's go over some of the most frequently asked questions when it comes to intermittent fasts. Here you will finally find all of the answers to your most bewildering of intermittent fast FAQs.

Will Intermittent Fasting Make Me Fat?

Although anyone who has read this book would have to know the answer to this question—let's just go over it here again, just for the sake of clarity. So, what's the answer? It's—no, absolutely not. Intermittent fasting does not make you fat, it helps you to burn fat. The whole structure of intermittent fasting is built around the idea of harnessing our unique physiologies so that we can make the most of metabolism and our body's natural ability to tap into fat deposits for energy.

While starvation diets will indeed lead to slower metabolisms and a possible increase in fat storage, intermittent fasting cuts through all that by keeping the body on an even keel. With intermittent fasting you essentially deprive the body of nutrients just enough to get it to burn extra surplus fat already in place—you then switch gears shortly thereafter back to standard nutrients so that there is no serious disruption in metabolism. So once again, let me assure those of you that may still have your doubts. Intermittent fasting won't make you fat, it will make you a lean, mean, fasting machine!

What's the best time to exercise during a fast?

We all have busy schedules, and we have to make our life work around them. Having that said, your own personal schedule is something that you should take into consideration when coupling a workout routine along with your fasting regimen. It's not good after all, to have two separate activities that compete with each other—

exercising and fasting. You need to have these two components complimenting each other rather than contrasting. Once you've got the timing hammered out, one of the key things to note, is that your body is at its most optimal for fat burn and muscle gain potential, between meals. So, if you are on the 12 day fast for example, you might want to exercise in the morning right after you have skipped breakfast, and then replenish your nutrient stores with either a late lunch or an early dinner. Whichever may work best for you at the time.

Would diet sodas be permissible during a fast?

Sorry folks, but the answer is no. I wish it weren't. Believe me, I love soda just as much as anyone else, but there isn't any arguing on this one. Diet sodas raise your insulin, and present the danger of increasing weight gain, even while you fast. It's like trying to put out a fire with a gallon of gasoline, it doesn't work. In other words, the sweeteners used in diet soda are a metabolic train wreck waiting to happen, and should be completely avoided during your fast.

Are there any initial negative reactions at the beginning of a fast?

I would be lying to you if I said that there was no difficulty or hardship experienced during an intermittent fast. The truth is, during the first couple days you may find yourself under some duress. Usually this presents itself in the form of a headache and slight fatigue. Some may even have the sensation that their body temperature has dropped, and feel like they have cold and clammy hands. As bad as this may sound, it's a sign that your body is working overtime to send blood to your fat tissue, warning it to prep itself for useable energy—in other words, that fat is getting ready to burn! Any feeling of discomfort during the process however, will quickly subside. And the long-term benefits will far outshine any short-term hardship.

Will I lose Muscle Mass during my Fast?

The answer to this one is rather straightforward. No, you are not likely to lose muscle during an intermittent fast. Even if you do not do any of the exercises recommended in this book, the fact that you are interspersing non-fasting regular meals in between your fast days should be enough to prevent any noticeable muscle loss. Weight training of course is another option to boost muscle, but really intermittent fasting should be enough to negate muscle loss.

Do you have to spend much money prepping for your Fast?

This is an excellent question and it's true that a lot of resource guides out there on intermittent fasting fail to properly address it. But the simple answer is—no. No, it's not going to cost you an arm and a leg to get the right ingredients to fast. In this book especially, we have made sure to use ingredients that most people could quite easily afford at their local grocery store. You don't have to shop for the most expensive organic foods. There isn't anything fancy in the meals and recipes presented in this book, just good, clean, affordable foods that are commonplace in most parts of the world.

Conclusion: Living Life in the Fast Lane

In many ways, a regimen of intermittent fasting is a call to action. It's a call to step out of the mundane and into the exciting. Rather than living a passive, sedentary life of caloric accumulation, intermittent fasting allows you to take charge of your own physiology. Intermittent fasting allows you to begin to literally dispose and dispense with the fat being stored in your body. There is something truly liberating about being able to take charge, and make use of your own natural metabolic drive in this fashion.

And if you have struggled with your weight in the past, this technique we call intermittent fasting, promises to be a true game changer. No longer are you at the mercy of your own fickle metabolism—you are in the driver's seat. By purposefully controlling when and what you eat you can choose how your body gets its energy. Intermittent fasting also kickstarts a self-healing and restorative process known as autophagy in which the body can replenish damaged and ineffective tissue at a much more rapid clip.

As you may have noticed, just about everything is sped up and more efficient during an intermittent fast. This is in stark contrast to the slow and barely noticeable weight loss that other more traditional low-calorie diets provide. Because trying to lose weight without the benefit of intermittent fasting is a lot like being stuck in traffic—you're trying hard to get to your destination but soon realize that you are going nowhere fast. But you don't have to wait any longer. Go ahead and take what you've learned here to heart, and get ready to start living your life in the fast lane! Thank you for reading!

If you liked this book—please leave me a review on Amazon to let me know about it. I really appreciate, and look forward to your feedback!

Download my FREE booklet: *Intermittent Fasting: 10 Simple & Healthy Recipes to Lose Weight & Get Healthy*
URL: https://forms.aweber.com/form/74/1929639774.htm

Amazon Author Page
URL: https://www.amazon.com/Silvia-Pala/e/B081F8SBBW/

Newsletter: subscribe to it TODAY to receive news, updates, recipes, free digital contents & much more on Intermittent Fasting!
URL: https://forms.aweber.com/form/43/890810243.htm

FB Group:
Please join my Facebook group to receive the latest updates, recipes, news and much more on intermittent fasting!

URL: https://www.facebook.com/groups/504409536885001/

Made in the USA
Monee, IL
23 September 2022